G-Spot Orgasm

Unleashing her
G-Spot Orgasm

A Step-by-Step Guide
to Achieving Ultimate Sexual Ecstasy

Donald L. Hicks

Amorata Press

Published by Amorata Press,
        an imprint of Ulysses Press
        P.O. Box 3440
        Berkeley, CA 94703
        www.amoratapress.com

Portions of this book were previously published under the title *Understanding the G-Spot and Female Sexuality*.

ISBN10: 1-56975-563-9
ISBN13: 978-1-56975-563-1
Library of Congress Control Number 2006903809

Editor: Lily Chou
Copyeditor: Mark Rhynsburger
Production: Matt Orendorff, Lisa Kester
Cover design: what!design @ whatweb.com
Cover photograph: ©iStockphoto.com

Printed in Canada by Webcom

10 9 8 7 6 5 4

Distributed by Publishers Group West

To Arleta,
the one person who has always encouraged me to write,
and has unwavering confidence in my abilities,
even when I lack faith in myself.

Contents

Preface

Greetings, reader!

Many years ago I, just like you, had questions about the G-spot. I wanted to know what the G-spot was, how to find it, and how to stimulate it. I also had a host of other questions similar to those you may be having today.

Back in that day, however, prior to the vast explosion of the Internet, there was a great lack of information available regarding the G-spot. On one hand, there were a couple of credible books on the subject, but these focused primarily on the medical aspects and existence of the G-spot rather than serving as a hands-on guide or Q & A book for the average Joe. At the opposite end of the spectrum were numerous G-spot stories in risqué or pornographic publications, yet these were often submitted anonymously and lacked authority or credibility.

As a freelance author accustomed to doing in-depth research, I was undaunted at the thought of finding answers to my questions. Little did I know, however, that what would start as "a few simple phone calls" would become a project spanning decades, eventually culminating in the first edition of this book and, now, in this revised and expanded edition.

My journey began by calling a few physicians with my questions. While some of my questions were answered efficiently, I was surprised to learn how many physicians were reluctant to discuss the G-spot, dismissed it entirely, or simply hadn't had the chance to study the latest research findings. (In defense of the latter, I can sincerely appreciate this since so many medical studies and findings are released each year—not just on the G-spot, but also on new drugs and studies of all parts of the body. It seems impossible for anyone to keep up.)

Still seeking answers to some of my questions, over a period of many months I was referred up the medical hierarchy. Each time one of my questions was answered, a new, more perplexing question would emerge, requiring another referral up the medical hierarchy. First I spoke to gynecologists, next to specialists, then to professors at medical schools, to experts at well-known institutions, and eventually to world-renowned leading experts and researchers—the very researchers who create the studies that are taught in medical school.

While determined to find answers, I must admit that when I was first referred to these big names, I was a bit intimidated. After all, throughout my climb up the medical hierarchy, I had heard echoes of their names. Who was I to interrupt them with my insignificant questions? In my mind, I envisioned them as stodgy, disdainful, presumptuous—each caught up in adding laurels to their already prestigious reputations—with no time for a non-Ph.D. such as myself, asking elementary questions. Of all the surprises I encountered along this journey, the biggest was finding out how mistaken this perception was. Not only were these "cream of the crop" researchers friendly, they were far from stodgy and were passionate about their work. Where I had envisioned them as disdainful, they were appreciative of my personal quest for knowledge and were willing to go out of their way to help me find answers. And where I had envisioned them as presumptuous, they were in fact very unselfish, placing more emphasis on seeing that correct knowledge got out rather than sticking a feather in their cap.

They were quick to share their knowledge and findings, willing to share their research, and helpful in directing me to the information I was seeking.

It was at about this point that the idea for this book was born. I recognized that despite the ben-

> *"I had a lot of misconceptions before I read this book. I thought I could always hit a woman's G-spot with my penis. Although it stings the ego, it's better to realize you were wrong than continue being wrong."* —L. J. T.

eficial intentions of these researchers to share their findings, much of this information wasn't trickling down to family physicians. Even less of it ever reached the general public. And here was I, an author privy to some of the most recent and pertinent research on the G-spot, someone able to serve as a conduit to bridge the communication gaps.

Over the next couple of years, I began privately developing the technique covered in this book, conducting surveys, gathering additional data, verifying my research, and making refinements. The finished product is what you now hold in your hands.

The purpose of this book is clear. It is a simple guide, backed with some of the latest modern research, yet written in layman's terms, without medical jargon. Its aim is to help couples around the world understand and enjoy the pleasures of the G-spot.

Read on. For now your own journey begins...

1

Learning the Basics

You may be wondering if the G-spot is real. Does it exist, or is all the G-spot hype just a selling tool for magazine articles or adult novelties? And if the G-spot does exist, why is it there? Why is it so easily overlooked? What physical purpose does it have? Does the penis come into contact with it during intercourse? How does one find it and coax it from hiding? This book will answer all these questions.

You may also wonder about female ejaculation—or *squirting*, as the phenomenon is often called. Is squirting merely so much more sales hype, or is female ejaculation real? And if female ejaculation does occur, why haven't you seen it? Why does it occur? What physical purpose is there for female ejaculation?

If you're pondering any of these questions, let me take a moment to congratulate you for taking the time to enrich your knowledge and understanding of female sexuality. As you'll learn from these pages, the phenomena of the G-spot and female ejaculation are not new. References to these enigmas can be traced back through history, from as early as the writings of Aristotle. As sad as it may seem, however, millions of people have lived and died, reaching their graves without ever experiencing the joys and pleasures offered by the G-spot (or seeing their partner thrash in the ecstasy of a G-spot orgasm).

The goal of this book is simple: to show you that G-spot orgasms and female ejaculation are real, they exist, and they can be evoked to bring about the ultimate in female ecstasy and sexual enjoyment. More important, you'll learn why these two phenomena exist, how they've been overlooked countless times in the past, and the important role they play in the processes of human reproduction and childbirth.

In these pages, you'll learn a proven ten-step technique that shows you how to find the G-spot, how to stimulate it, and how to drive your lover crazy with ecstasy. You'll deepen your understanding of the female anatomy while learning new methods of rekindling the romance and sexual excitement in your current relationship.

The G-spot does exist, and through this book, you can prove it to yourself. And your lover.

What's the Big Deal about G-Spot Orgasms, Anyway?

"My lover and I already have great sex. Why do we need to worry about the G-spot?"

If you've never seen or experienced a true G-spot orgasm, imagine for a moment an orgasm that causes the whole vagina to spasm violently, often contracting so tightly that it tries to force out your finger or any object in the vagina. And imagine that while these intense contractions are throbbing and pulsing throughout the vagina, the vagina becomes very wet, often literally ejaculating a stream or spurt of fluid with each contraction. Imagine an orgasm that causes such intense ecstasy that even the quietest and most controlled woman will yelp and buck and thrash, while normal "screamers" go dead silent, the scream caught in their throat—a scream that if freed might wake all the neighbors within a five-block radius.

Want more reasons? Here's another favorable point to consider: Have you ever had sex and afterward wondered, "Did she really orgasm, or was that an Oscar performance for my benefit?" I think it's safe to say that most men encounter this distasteful "Did she fake it?" uncertainty at one time or another. Now imagine an orgasm with no guesswork or worries about faking. Imagine an orgasm that provides you with *clear physical signs* that occur involuntarily. No doubt. No guesswork. This is the glory of a G-spot orgasm.

But don't take my word for it alone. Here's what a few others had to say:

> *"I didn't think orgasms like that were real . . . I thought they only existed in romance novels."* —B. R.

> *"It was absolutely the deepest, most wonderful climax I've ever felt! It was like warmth started in my very center and flowed outward all over my body. I loved it!"* —L. K.

> *"I thought I had wet the bed! And then [name withheld] explained what had happened and I could hardly*

believe it finally happened to me. If I have to wash the sheets every day for the rest of my life, it's worth it."
—T. J.

"I wanted it to last forever, and couldn't stand another second . . . both at the same time. It was the greatest!"
—M. J. J.

"After that, I'll never let [name withheld] get away from me! Our love life has never been better." —K. A.

"She used to just lie there and moan through the whole thing. It was frustrating because I never knew when she was orgasming or if she even orgasmed. Thanks to your technique, there's no more guessing." —T. P.

The Dire Truth about Conventional Orgasms

While most men can go from "slightly interested" to "full ejaculation" in an average of three to four minutes, orgasms for women are often more elusive. On average, a woman requires 15 minutes (or longer) of combined foreplay and stimulation before orgasm is achieved. The reward: a clitoral or vaginal orgasm lasting an average of 8 to 19 seconds.

In the early 1970s, *The Hite Report*, a detailed nationwide study, determined that nearly 12 percent of women never experienced any type of orgasm. The same study discovered that 16 percent could have an orgasm during intercourse (with the addition of clitoral stimulation) and 19 percent achieved a rare orgasm through intercourse alone.

Only 26 percent had an orgasm on a regular basis (30 percent when including those who claimed to have vague "good feelings" in the vagina). Couple this with the brief 8-to-19-second duration of an average orgasm and you have a very dire picture.

Another segment of the study showed controversy over "clitoral orgasms" versus "vaginal orgasms." The consensus revealed that clitoral orgasms (empty vagina) were largely considered "higher intensity" than orgasms with vaginal penetration.

But there was a catch. During clitoral stimulation and orgasm, most women felt a strong desire to have an object in the vagina, and often craved "thrusting" within the vagina. The problem with this "vaginal craving" was that there was an immediate decrease in pleasure if vaginal penetration was made.

Additional parts of *The Hite Report* concluded that orgasm intensities could range from questionable ("Was that an orgasm I felt?") to pure ecstasy, but the high-intensity orgasms occurred much less frequently. The study also showed that most women have intercourse for the purpose of sharing emotional intimacy, while another group's primary motivation was to obtain the ever-elusive orgasm. One part of the study revealed that about a third of the women studied enjoyed anal penetration while another third didn't like anal penetration. Another section ascertained that 21 percent of women desired daily sex, while 18 percent—nearly the same amount—were satisfied with sex three times per week. Other studies in *The Hite Report* considered masturbation with fingers versus objects, sex with the legs together versus spread, and the preference for different positions during sex.

This information only serves to underline the obvious: Each of us is different in a wide variety of ways. While one person enjoys drinking coffee, another may not. And while one person enjoys having their partner blow into their ear, another may find the sensation unpleasant. While one person enjoys having their partner suck their toes, another finds the act disgusting. While one woman may be turned on (even to orgasm) by having her breasts fondled and nuzzled, another may find breast stimulation undesirable.

Because everyone likes and dislikes different things, it's important to communicate openly with your partner and share what both of you really enjoy—and what you don't. Talk to each other and let your partner know what turns you on and what doesn't.

The study results cited above also elucidate the sad reality that many women never orgasm, and that those who do aren't always satisfied afterward. But now there is hope.

Not only do many women report G-spot orgasms to be highly satisfying, but the duration of a G-spot orgasm is considerably longer than the normal vaginal or clitoral orgasm. The G-spot orgasm often lasts *45 seconds*—with common reports of two-minute orgasms and rare reports of orgasms lasting between 20 and 40 minutes! One man reported:

> *"She kept orgasming as long as I was rubbing the spot.*
> *It never quit or slowed down. We have a clock radio on*
> *our night table and it went on for at least 45 minutes.*
> *I know that sounds like an exaggeration, but it's not. I*

*was beginning to think it might harm her in some
way if I kept going. And I was ready to explode any
minute. Watching her thrash around in ecstasy and
feeling how warm and wet her [vagina] was against
my fingers was driving me crazy. Her [vagina] kept
contracting and squeezing and she felt as tight as a
schoolgirl again. It was driving me crazy. I love this
G-spot thing."*

A few women have reported needing to stop their partners
from continuing stimulation because the pleasure was "excruciating" or "nearly unbearable." One woman stated:

*"The anxiety was overwhelming. At first I thought it
would never come and when it did, the ecstasy was
almost unbearable. It felt so wonderful I couldn't stand
it. I thought I might go crazy from the pleasure. I
wanted to keep going, but had to stop, both at the
same time. And when it was over, I was exhausted
and totally satiated. Total bliss doesn't define what I
felt. It's not even close."*

Beyond driving your lover crazy with long-lasting ecstasy,
an additional benefit of G-spot stimulation may be a reduction in risk for cancer and diseases in the female prostate
(also known as the Skene's glands, or the paraurethral glands
and ducts). While the occurrence of female prostate cancer
is low and it is seldom fatal, any reduction of risk is still
beneficial. According to many alternative health experts
and Eastern practices, massaging the prostate can drain toxins and stress. In the book *The Prostate Miracle: New Natural*

Therapies That Can Save Your Life,[1] the authors discuss similar means for cleansing the male prostate gland and releasing toxins. Although the female prostate is smaller than the male counterpart, the two develop from the same embryonic tissue. Because of their similarity, one might hypothesize that stimulation of the female prostate and the corollary release of fluids and cleansing could offer the same benefits to women. This topic of women's health deserves future research.

The 92 Percent Factor

Using the technique provided in this book, an astounding 92 percent of our respondents reported success within the first three applications of the technique. This percentage includes women who previously considered themselves either "nonorgasmic" or reported low occurrences of orgasm.

While that might not sound impressive at first, consider this: Assuming this statistic were to hold true, if you have 100 women who are sexually active and who may have had sex hundreds of times before without ever experiencing an orgasm, 92 of the 100 would experience a G-spot orgasm within the first three applications of this technique. That's pretty impressive.

In one survey I conducted, women were instructed to grade or rate vaginal, clitoral, and G-spot orgasms on a scale of 1 to 10 (with 10 being "most pleasurable" and 1 being "least pleasurable"). Of the respondents who achieved successful G-spot orgasms, the average rating was 10. (Several even claimed it was "off the chart.") In the same study, the average clitoral orgasm was rated 8 and vaginal orgasms ranked third in pleasure intensity, with an average rating of 6.

When asked to describe their G-spot orgasm experience, women commonly made these four comments:

"It was deeper than anything I'd felt before."

"It felt very different from previous orgasms."

"It was more fulfilling/satisfying than previous orgasms."

"It felt better/more pleasurable/more intense than other orgasms I've had."

In addition, many women equated the G-spot orgasm to a "whole body" event, whereas other orgasms were "pelvic." Many comments also referenced feeling a "heat" that "started deep within the core" and spread throughout the body. Coinciding with this statement, many of the sexual partners who administered the technique made comments such as "She broke out in a sweat afterward" or "She was drenched and exhausted" or, more simply, "She threw off the covers." Many women also reported that their first (observed) female ejaculation occurred with the G-spot orgasm. One recurring comment was "I thought I'd wet the bed."

While G-spot orgasms and female ejaculations are separate entities, the two sometimes occur simultaneously. I'll discuss female ejaculation later, in detail.

Like finding a half-bloomed rose, you now have a glimpse of the G-spot's glory. Soon the petals will unfold.

Why Does the G-Spot Exist?

Beyond the intense sexual pleasure the G-spot is able to produce, new studies are investigating the G-spot's value in blocking pain during childbirth. In an article titled "Beyond the G Spot: Recent Research on Female Sexuality"[2] that appeared in the January 1999 issue of *Psychiatric Annals*, authors Beverly Whipple and Barry Komisaruk stated: ". . . a series of studies has demonstrated that self-stimulation of the anterior wall of the vagina in women produces a significant elevation in pain thresholds" and "we believe childbirth would be more painful without this natural pain-blocking effect."

This research, which has since been replicated by other researchers, reveals the G-spot's significance during childbirth. It is now believed that the two physical purposes of the G-spot are 1) to ease pain during childbirth (as shown by Whipple and Komisaruk), and 2) to enhance or provide sexual pleasure.

When I say "enhancing sexual pleasure," I am referring to indirect G-spot stimulation. For example, when the penis swells during normal intercourse, the increased girth of the penis may partially stimulate the G-spot and "boost" or accelerate a woman's sexual enjoyment, often to the point that she orgasms with her partner. If your female lover has ever said anything like "You started swelling and hitting something up in there that felt great," you now understand what was happening. Likely, the partial stimulation of the G-spot enhanced her sexual pleasure, and possibly accelerated her orgasm.

When I say "providing sexual pleasure," I am referring to direct stimulation of the G-spot, which, as you'll soon learn, can provide a standalone, unparalleled source of orgasm.

A Side Order to Go, Please

By following the technique outlined in this book, you can reap many direct rewards. In addition, there are also indirect rewards along the way. The ten-step system is designed to teach G-spot understanding and prowess, yet it also incorporates the building blocks for enriching and strengthening relationships.

Heightened intimacy is a good example. We all need a partner with whom we can share our hopes and dreams, our fears and desires, our failures and our triumphs. We need some-

> *"I love seeing my wife in a teddy, a garter, thigh-highs, and high heels. I'm a leg and breast man and that ensemble is a real turn-on for me. However, before I learned your technique, I had to beg my wife to dress up for me in her 'play clothes.' Now she meets me at the door in her 'play clothes' every day after work. Thank you."* —D. L.

one to laugh with and someone to help us forget the pressures society heaps on our shoulders. Sharing intimacy and having friends to confide in can be an important element of not only a strong relationship but also good emotional health: a "side order."

The spontaneous praise that results from the ten-step program is another suitable example. When we're dating that special someone, praise is a wonderful tool. It's a great way to elicit a smile, a word of thanks, or perhaps even a kiss. We use praise to suggest our feelings toward that person by saying "I love *this* about you" or "I love *that* about you." And because of the smile it often evokes, we freely point out our mate's beauties, skills, or whatever qualities we admire in them. They smile, love us for our admiration, and often return a similar sentiment.

As the relationship progresses, however, and simmers, we tend to withdraw from praising our partner. In return, our partner withdraws from praising us. Offering praise becomes similar to giving part of ourselves away, a silent forfeiture of power. It fosters feelings of inadequacy and somehow makes us feel as if we're "less" and the other person "more." Beyond that, the lack of received praise begins to gnaw at our own self-worth. We start second-guessing whether our partner still admires the traits she or he once freely applauded. We wonder if we still please them in bed. We vow not to venture out on a shaky limb and praise our partner if they no longer praise us. The same praise we once used as a helpful tool that frequently led to the bedroom now has become a barrier. We have set ourselves up for a "praise standoff" with our mate, like two petulant children pretending to be gunslingers.

With the stealth of a snake, a rift has split the ground between us and our partner, widening with the passage of time until we are separated by an immense void.

But this need not be the case. As we know, the world can be a harsh place. It continually beats us down and, at times, the simplest word of encouragement from our mate can bolster and fortify us, giving us the strength to lift our chin and carry on. By recognizing the fact that we benefit from receiving praise, it's easy to understand that our mate can benefit in all the same ways. And whom do we want to be the source of our mate's praise: ourselves, or a stranger? What does it really cost us to give praise? What might it cost if we don't?

Like most things worthy of pursuit, the rewards that you and your partner receive along the way to the G-spot—pleasure, tenderness, open communication, increased sexual awareness and sexual expression—will reflect the effort you extend.

Consider what one successful user of the technique had to say:

> *"Thanks so much for introducing me to the G-spot and sharing your wealth of sexual know-how. You have no idea how beneficial your time and insightful comments have been in restoring my marriage. Before reading your book, my wife and I were on the brink of separating. Lovemaking had become an unimaginative weekly ritual for us. The fires of romance that once blazed brightly had dwindled to a pile of cool ashes. We spoke to each other only out of necessity and both felt we had grown apart. Now that has changed. The knowledge you imparted has changed that. By following your suggested steps, the doors of communication reopened. My wife and I discovered that we still have many common goals; they were just buried underneath the headaches of everyday life. We were both bored in the bedroom and had little desire to cuddle or do anything that might lead to sex. Now, we're like teenage lovers again. Our relationship is renewed. We take walks together,*

talk openly, and have adventurous sex daily (twice if we can manage). It all started that first night I tried your technique. The seed for new growth was planted. I (we) can't thank you enough."—G. P.

If your relationship has grown stale and lacks romantic luster, congratulate yourself for purchasing this book. You've taken a positive step toward rekindling the fires of romance. And while buying a book may seem insignificant, remember that knowledge is a powerful tool. Sometimes the tiniest of sparks can set off the largest inferno.

The matches are now in your hand.

Blended Orgasms: A Recipe for Higher Ecstasy

Suppose for a moment that your mate mentally rates a clitoral orgasm as a 7 and a G-spot orgasm as a 10. What would happen if she felt both of these orgasms at the same time? The answer is simple: She would experience a blended orgasm—something right off the chart!

In the early 1970s, Dr. Irving Singer touched upon the concept of "blended orgasms."[3] Thereafter, while studying the continuum of orgasmic response and the corresponding nerve pathways, Drs. Beverly Whipple, Alice Kahn Ladas, and John Perry validated, defined, and clarified the reality of blended orgasms.[4]

In layman's terms, blended orgasms are "two or more orgasms occurring simultaneously (or in very close rotation)." Blended orgasms originate from multiple sources of simulation. For example, if you perform cunnilingus as you stimulate your partner's G-spot, she may experience a blended clitoral/G-spot orgasm.

While the two obvious sources for blended orgasms are 1) stimulation of the clitoris and G-spot and 2) stimulation of the clitoris and vagina, we need not limit our thinking to these two combinations. An orgasm can originate from a variety of sources. For some women, having their breasts massaged or nuzzled is very pleasurable and can bring about orgasm. For others, petting and necking (with or without breast stimulation) can induce an orgasm. Others reported orgasms occurring during dreams, while horseback-riding, and even while dancing.[5] And for others, mental imagery alone (without any physical stimulation)[6,7] can cultivate orgasm.

Unlike the fortunate women who can orgasm easily, 12 percent of women, as discussed earlier, reported never experiencing any type of orgasm. Others reported being able to orgasm only through one type of stimulation, such as clitoral. Logic would therefore indicate that not all women are likely to experience blended orgasms—unless they find new sources or methods of becoming orgasmic.

While it is only a pet theory awaiting further research, I believe that women who are skilled multitaskers, those who commonly engage in two or more activities at once, are more likely to experience blended orgasms. This is because orgasming is largely a choice, processed and occurring in the brain.

To Orgasm or Not to Orgasm?

This is the question many people ask themselves during intercourse. It's my hope and goal that you enjoy the benefit of seeing your mate experience a blended orgasm. And, it warrants mentioning here, your display of unselfishness and caring is commendable. However, while the thought of seeing your mate experience a blended orgasm may be appealing, you must learn to walk before you can run.

It is important, first of all, to understand and accept that people choose to have an orgasm. Deciding to orgasm is a mental choice. No one can "give" or "will" another person an orgasm, or "make" them orgasm, no more than you can "will" a stranger to remove their clothing. We can create an environment and ambience favorable for orgasm: We can dim the lights, set out the candles, put on music, and spread sweet rose petals. We can also provide physical and emotional stimulation. But ultimately, the choice "to orgasm or not to orgasm" is the individual's.

Often, without consciously deliberating, each of us makes individual choices concerning "if" or "when" we will achieve orgasm. For those who are highly orgasmic, the sheer act of removing clothing (or allowing it to be removed) may mark the decision to orgasm: the unconscious "yes." For others, however, the decision may not be made until they have tested the waters and stimulation or coitus is under way, often mere seconds before the orgasm explodes onto the scene. Others release their reservations in layers. Like an autumn tree shedding its leaves, they slowly drop their inhibitions as they grow more secure, comfortable, and relaxed with the situation. Yet some others refuse to ever relinquish control, usually from fear of self-humiliation, from insecurity with the relationship, or to avoid appearing too "wanton" or "loose."

There are several determining factors in making the decision whether and when to have an orgasm. In order to "let go" and orgasm, most people need to feel secure with their partner, first and foremost. We also need to feel good about ourselves, safe in our chosen location, relaxed, and comfortable with what's happening to our bodies.

One woman aptly compared a fulfilling romantic encounter to a multiple-course meal:

> *"There are times when it's okay to just have a snack. A snack can stave off the hunger pangs and get you through a moment, but a snack is never totally fulfilling, and always leaves you wanting more. If you really want to orgasm and be fulfilled and satiated afterward, you need the whole meal . . . the full course. You need an appetizer of romantic foreplay to feel confident that your partner really cares about you, doesn't want to just get in your pants, isn't going disappear before morning and be out describing your body to his buddies, and won't embarrass you by talking about private acts that took place in the bedroom. You need to feel loved. You also need the meat and potatoes of security and time, knowing that someone isn't going to walk in on you, or one of you isn't going to have to jump up and rush out to work at an inopportune moment. A side dish of relaxation can also help, so your mind isn't constantly reminding you of what errands you need to accomplish, what bills need to be paid, and other worries that can interrupt the mood. (Have you ever tried to get in the mood when you have a hundred things to do?)*

*Most importantly, you need the dessert of love and
romance—knowing that you and your partner love
each other, want to pleasure each other, are willing
to stop if it's needed, and will be together next month
and next year.*

*If you want to be really fulfilled afterward, it takes the
whole meal. A snack just won't do."*

As you may recall, one of the four most common descriptions of the G-spot experience I receive is "It felt very different from previous orgasms." Keep this in mind. At some point while you're applying the G-spot technique, your partner may realize that something new and very exciting is happening to her. And that is the moment when she will decide whether to orgasm or not to orgasm.

There are pros and cons to telling your mate beforehand of your plans to administer the G-spot technique. If you tell her, you may set her up to be a victim of "orgasm anxiety" (discussed on page 75). On the other hand, if she senses that something new and unknown is happening to her as you apply the technique, she may delay or inhibit her orgasm due to the uncertainty and novelty of what she's feeling.

I'd personally recommend that you don't initially mention your plan to administer the technique. Instead, watch for signs of uncertainty as she senses that this is something new. When you see these signs, begin reassuring her that you know what's occurring and understand it. "I know what's happening to you. It's okay. I'm here, just enjoy what you feel."

The same thinking applies to blended orgasms. While the pursuit of blended orgasms is encouraged, don't overwhelm her by trying to make the first G-spot orgasm a blended G-spot/clitoral orgasm. Take it one step at a time. After she becomes familiar with G-spot experiences, gaining both confidence and understanding, she'll be better suited (if not eager) to explore the bold world of blended orgasms.

Intimacy 101

Merriam-Webster's defines the word *intimate* as:

> *"Marked by very close association, contact, or familiarity; marked by a warm friendship; suggesting informal warmth or privacy; of a very private and personal nature."*

As this definition suggests, people share intimacy not only with their lovers or sexual partners but also with close friends, family members, and even pets. Since the subject matter of this book deals with the intracouple relationship, most references to intimacy here relate to the bonding, the private and personal sharing, and the carnal aspects of relationships.

It's important to acknowledge that intimacy need not be linked to sex. Intimacy is the sharing of one's innermost feelings and thoughts with someone we trust. Not only does intimacy create a temporary buffer to the outside world, it also provides a brief respite from stress. It staves off loneliness and promotes self-worth. While conversations take place from mind to mind, intimacy occurs from heart to heart.

The Phenomenon of Female Ejaculation

Before we move on, let's take a moment to explore the subject of female ejaculation. Modern society fosters the myth that G-spot orgasms and female ejaculation are the *same occurrence*. While the two do often occur together, it's important to realize that they are *separate wonders*—not one entity.

When this book was first released, I served as a voluntary advisor on several Internet forums, including for the Oxygen cable TV network program *Talk Sex with Sue* and forums at alt.sex. All too often, a recurring situation would play out. It would begin with a female poster arriving at the boards, describing her first (observed) female ejaculation and asking if anyone knew what it was—was it normal, should she see a doctor, etc. Invariably, four or five people would promptly respond, telling her, "You've just had your first G-spot orgasm!"

As you will learn, while G-spot orgasms and female ejaculation often occur simultaneously, either one can occur without the other. Here are answers to some of the most common questions about female ejaculation:

If G-spot orgasms and female ejaculation aren't the same, what exactly is "female ejaculation"?

Female ejaculation occurs when a women "ejaculates" fluid (different from urine, but possibly containing urine) from her urethra during sexual arousal or orgasm. While it may accompany a G-spot or other orgasm, female ejaculation has been observed to occur without any stimulation to the G-spot.

Where does this fluid come from?

Surrounding the urethra and running to the neck of the bladder lie a network of glands, ducts, and nerves called the Skene's glands or the paraurethral glands. As mentioned earlier, these glands are the female counterparts to the male prostrate. The Skene's glands are the source of female ejaculate.

If it's not urine, what is this fluid?

The fluid is typically described as "clear" or "milky," having little or no odor, and often having a sweet taste. However, as with male secretion, the taste may change due to dietary intake or possibly as part of the menstruation cycle.[8] Additionally, while I am not aware of any sound medical research on the subject, it is often rumored that drinking pineapple juice can sweeten the taste of both female and male ejaculations, and may also increase their volume. Since pineapple juice is high in fructose and glucose, the rumor would appear to have some legitimacy.

What is the chemical makeup of the ejaculate?

The primary chemical makeup of the fluid is glucose, fructose, prostate specific antigen (PSA) and prostatic acid phosphatase (PAP).[9,10,11,12] The fluid may also contain traces of urine.[13] Interestingly enough, fructose is one of the components present in male ejaculation. Its primary job is to mobilize the spermatozoa. While it was once believed that male fructose was the sole propellant of spermatozoa, the presence of fructose in female ejaculate provides evidence to the contrary. Instead of passively waiting for spermatozoa to "swim" to the egg, the female plays an active role in the insemination process by infusing her own fructose to usher the spermatozoa toward their goal, thus increasing the probability for successful fertilization.

Because of this, it is believed that the physical purpose of female ejaculation is to aid in the mobilization of spermatozoa. And while it may not be scientifically proven, it stands to reason that stimulation of the G-spot and the female prostate may be a beneficial pursuit for couples facing problems with conception.

> "The first time she came, it looked like she was about to give birth. She hunched forward and all this fluid shot out of her and splattered on my arm. I didn't believe in the G-spot until that moment. Believe me, it's real." —I. J. S.

On a related subject, early forensic medicine mandated the checking of rape victims, and the spots on their clothing, for the presence of acid phosphatase, to prove that rape had occurred. Research on female ejaculate has since proven this test has no forensic value, since female ejaculation also contains acid phosphatase.

What causes female ejaculation?

Since the G-spot resides near the Skene's glands, and the glands are often caressed during G-spot stimulation, fluid is often released into the urethra as a result of G-spot stimulation. However, G-spot stimulation is not the sole source of ejaculation. Some women have been observed to ejaculate with stimulation of the clitoris alone.[14,15]

Do all women ejaculate?

Evidence is inconclusive as to whether all women have the ability to ejaculate. If the presence of fructose is designed to play an important role in reproduction, one might hypothesize that all women would have the ability to ejaculate (excluding those with physical anomalies, of course, or surgical removal of the Skene's glands, disease, or hereditary disorders). Nonetheless, researchers in some studies of healthy women observed no expulsion of fluid during stimulation.

In his *Secrets of Sensual Lovemaking: The Ultimate in Female Ecstasy*, Tom Leonardi states: ". . . a combination of physical technique and psychological security were absolutely necessary in order for a woman to have ejaculatory orgasms." Many of the accounts in Leonardi's book indicate the need for a strong emotional bond to be established prior to successful female ejaculation.[16] If this is true, it could explain why some laboratory studies fail whereas others, conducted in a more natural atmosphere, often succeed, especially those conducted by researchers who willingly provide in-home examination or testing. As I will demonstrate in the ten-step technique, emotional bonding is indeed a key ingredient to success.

It has also been hypothesized that, because many women are in a reclining position during intercourse or stimulation, the fluid is retroejaculated into the bladder and is later released during urination. In *The G Spot and Other Discoveries About Human Sexuality*, by Ladas, Whipple, and Perry, the authors state: "Some women may experience retrograde ejaculation if the fluid shoots into the bladder rather than out the urethra."[17] This condition might be characterized by a woman feeling the need to urinate after orgasm, but, when she tries to do so, only releasing a small amount of clear or milky fluid.

Dr. Francesco Cabello, author of "Female Ejaculation, Myth or Reality,"[18] tested the hypothesis that all women ejaculate and found that some may retrograde ejaculate and therefore might be unaware of the ejaculation, since the fluid becomes mixed with urine in the bladder and is later released during urination.

Of the 212 completed and usable surveys I received in doing research for this guide, 48 percent of the female respondents reported that they did not ejaculate or were unsure if they had ejaculated. At the other end of the spectrum, 5 percent reported ejaculating before orgasm and 47 percent reported ejaculating during G-spot orgasm. Of the 110 women who reported ejaculating, 101 reported that the incident was their first known ejaculation. Eight others stated that they had ejaculated in the past, while one woman informed us that she commonly ejaculates with stimulation of the breasts, clitoris, and vagina.

A 37-year-old woman reported:

> *"The first time I slept with [name withheld], I thought I'd wet the bed. It was very embarrassing for me because I really loved him and wanted sex to be good for us. And it was good in ways I'd never dreamed of. I've been having orgasms regularly since I was 16, but*

> *nothing like this had ever happened. I've slept with*
> *seven different men and always considered my sex life*
> *as 'good' until this orgasm. Now I know what I was*
> *missing all those years. This orgasm was very different*
> *and so much deeper and better than the ones I've had*
> *before. [name withheld] is a definite keeper."*

Another woman reported:

> *"I didn't know I could ejaculate. I'd heard of other*
> *women ejaculating but had no idea that I could do it*
> *until my friend applied your technique. It was quite*
> *an experience."*

Does the ejaculation always occur along with orgasm?

No. In a study conducted by M. Zaviacic et al. in 1998,[19] a group of ten women who ejaculate through G-spot stimulation were studied. Of the ten women, they found that two participants ejaculated within the first one and a half minutes of stimulation, prior to orgasm. Five other participants ejaculated after four to eight minutes of G-spot stimulation (again, prior to orgasm). And the three remaining participants ejaculated with orgasm, after 10 to 15 minutes of G-spot stimulation.

How much fluid is ejaculated?

This is a controversial topic. Most scientific studies gauge the average female ejaculation as "a few drops to one teaspoonful"—comparable to the average volume of semen ejaculated by males. In *The G Spot and Other Discoveries About Human Sexuality* (recommended reading), the authors state: "In the cases of female ejaculation observed by Whipple,

Perry, and their colleagues, only a few drops to about a quarter of a teaspoon were usually expelled."[20]

At the other end of the spectrum, I have received reports of women "drenching the bed" or producing "copious amounts" of fluid. One man had this to say:

"She left a wet circle about a foot in diameter. We were both amazed at how large the spot was. The sheets were saturated. There was no foul odor. No noticeable odor in fact. But the bed was too drenched to allow comfortable sleep."

Another man said:

"Sometimes it just trickles out of her and sometimes it gushes and leaves a big wet spot. It's great if she's on top because having that warm liquid flow down over my testicles makes me [ejaculate] almost instantly. We don't mind changing the sheets afterward. It's worth it."

Another stated:

"This milky liquid squirted out of her and splattered between her knees. It left a two-foot long wet streak on the sheets."

And:

"She normally ejaculates between one-half cup to one cup. But the first time [she ejaculated] it was more, maybe a cup and a half."

And:

"About a week after we started using your technique, we bought a plastic mattress liner for our bed. You might

> *want to recommend this to other people, along with buy-*
> *ing a couple of extra sets of sheets. Otherwise, the center*
> *of the bed gets too wet after a couple nights of fun."*

And:

> *"She literally drenched the bed. When it comes to*
> *volume, women put men to shame."*

A woman stated:

> *"I don't mind washing the wet bedclothes every day.*
> *This orgasm is worth it."*

In Tom Leonardi's *Secrets of Sensual Lovemaking, The Ultimate in Female Ecstasy*, several of the interview subjects indicated "large amounts of the fluid." On page 114 of the edition I've cited, one subject stated: "And the insides of her thighs were dripping wet." Another said: "She came and she squirted. It hit me in the arm. It hit my arm and I'm not sure where the rest of it went...from my forearm all the way up near my elbow."

In describing the event, Leonardi states on page 57: "At the very least, her hot liquid will quickly seep out of her, running down her buttocks and off her body. But most likely, the liquid will physically fly from her vagina—2, 4, 8, even 12 or more inches from her."

The "larger volume" conjecture might also be supported by a custom called *kachapati*, which was practiced by the Batoro tribe of Uganda, Africa. According to a personal communication from anthropologist Phil Kilbraten,[21] the *kachapati* was a rite of passage for young women emerging from puberty into womanhood. Before these young women were eligible for marriage, the older women of the village taught them how to ejaculate. The term *kachapati* literally means to "spray the walls." One might conclude that, in order to "spray the walls," a significant amount of fluid would need to be expelled.

So how is it that skilled researchers report only a "teaspoonful" or less while many people claim it's more?

Considering that most female ejaculations occur in dimly lit or near-dark conditions and are coupled with the excitement of lovemaking (and perhaps the novelty of a first-time event), I feel that some estimates of the fluid amount are exaggerated or overestimated. As a comparison, if you take a teaspoon of water and dump it onto a flat nonabsorbent surface, the water will form a circle approximately 3.5 inches in diameter. If you repeat the same experiment, but cover the hard surface with an absorbent piece of material (such as a cotton bedsheet), the teaspoon of water will soak outward and form a circle 8 inches in diameter. Since many mattresses are treated with stain-resistant protections such as Scotchgard and are covered with heavy upholstery that resists permeation, the bed linens often absorb (and diffuse) the bulk of the liquid. Also, because air can travel through the weave of many bed linens, the heat quickly dissipates and causes the area to feel cool and saturated.

Some researchers feel that urinary stress incontinence (USI) may also play a role, as urine is sometimes released "as" or "along with" ejaculate, thus increasing the volume. However, other researchers argue against this, claiming that because it is physiologically impossible for a man to urinate at the moment of orgasm, the same likely holds true for women. (This latter argument does not account for women ejaculating urine prior to orgasm.)

What does it all mean?

While the jury is still out on certain aspects of female ejaculation, advancing research has played a valuable role in the advancement and betterment of women's health. In the past, many women who described "ejaculations" to their physicians were misdiagnosed with USI and were often directed to undergo "corrective surgery" for the "problem." Beyond the embarrassment brought on by their "shameful condition," some women faced the wrath of a spouse who believed his wife urinated on him during intercourse! As one can see, the plight of these women was unpleasant. Fortunately, due to groundbreaking research by Addiego, Holoman, Komisaruk, Molcan, Perry, Whipple, Zaviacic, Zaviaciova, and other great researchers, acceptance of female ejaculation is coming about.

Some Healthy Considerations

Most medical doctors agree that the therapeutic values of intercourse far outweigh the risks, provided safer sex practices are followed. During intercourse, muscles can be exercised. Stress, stored in the muscle tissue, is released from the body. In addition, the physical stimulation and movement during both foreplay and intercourse force the heart to beat faster and breathing to increase. This causes oxygen-enriched blood to spread throughout the body, replenishing cells and feeding muscles.

We've all likely heard the office-water-cooler comment that so-and-so "must have gotten lucky last night" because he or she seems to glow and is unusually cheerful. These statements may have medical validity since, like all forms of exercise, the release of stress can brighten our disposition and help make the world less gloomy and foreboding.

When engaging in intercourse, readers are urged to practice safer sex. If you're not familiar with safer sex practices, there are a host of informative books available, such as *Safe Encounters: How Women Can Say "Yes" to Pleasure and "No" to Unsafe Sex* (Beverly Whipple and Gina Ogden, McGraw-Hill, 1989) or *Safe Sex in a Dangerous World* (Art Ulene, Vintage Books, 1987). Your family physician is also a good learning source. Many physicians have educational pamphlets available or can provide information on sexually transmitted diseases (STDs) and their avoidance.

Contrary to popular belief, the risk of heart attack occurring during sexual activity is very low. In a study performed with patients who have suffered heart problems,[22] only .09 percent cited sexual activity as the triggering factor. The energy consumed during sexual orgasm has been compared to "about the same energy required for climbing two flights of stairs . . . or walking on a treadmill at 3 to 4 miles per hour."[23] Compared to many other activities, the risk is low.

If you have a history of heart-related illnesses or other medical conditions such as blood pressure or blood sugar irregularities, you should check with your physician to learn safe guidelines. Also, know your partner's health. It's a wise practice to discuss his/her health status, including any sexual diseases and any other health concerns, before engaging in intercourse.

A Brief History of the G-Spot

There's an adage that states: "To know where you're going, it's helpful to know where you've been." This statement holds true for the G-spot. By cultivating a deeper knowledge and understanding of the G-spot's history, you increase your odds for success while using the ten-step technique.

We owe a great debt to the visionaries of our world. Not only to those who live today, but to those who have come and gone. Throughout time, gallant individuals have seen beyond common perceptions and silently shouldered the duty of discovering truth. In many cases, after enduring countless hours of research to validate their cause, these selfless individuals stepped forth buoyantly to declare their findings—only to have their hopes bludgeoned by ridiculing peers.

Christopher Columbus might serve as a fitting example. At age 14, he became a sailor. For many years, he studied known maps of the world; likely doubting the world was flat, as was commonly believed. Later, as his theories of a "round world" manifested themselves, he conferred with European scholars (who also believed the world was round). Gaining conviction, he set forth to prove his theory. Yet when he announced plans to sail to the East Indies by crossing the Atlantic toward the west, he was persecuted by "flat thinking" peers.

As we all know, Columbus sailed and prevailed. His ship did not fall off the edge of a flat Earth and into oblivion. And although he never reached his original destination, he discovered something greater in the process—a bold new uncharted world.

Like most great discoveries, the G-spot and the reality of female ejaculation follow a similar history. Throughout history, brave and dutiful visionaries have arisen time after time to confirm the existence of this uncharted sexual continent, often bearing the ridicule of skeptical peers in the process. Aristotle may be one of the earliest recorded observers to note that women expel fluid during orgasm. In the seventeenth century, a Dutch anatomist, Regnier de Graaf, described "female 'prostatae' or corpus glandulosum" which expulsed fluid, enhanced libido, and caused pleasure. In his findings, he stated: "The function of the 'prostatae' is to generate pituitoserous juice which makes women more libidinous" and "the discharge from the female 'prostatae' causes as much pleasure as does that from the male 'prostatae.'"[24]

Long after Regnier de Graaf's work, Alexander Skene, M.D., George Caldwell, M.D., John W. Huffman, M.D., Samuel Berkow, M.D., and several others individually studied these glands and the subject of female ejaculation and released their own findings.

At the end of World War II, a German gynecologist and obstetrician named Ernst Gräfenberg collaborated with an American gynecologist and obstetrician by the name of Robert L. Dickinson, M.D. In 1950, Gräfenberg wrote that "an erotic zone could always be demonstrated on the anterior wall of the vagina along the course of the urethra."[25] According to the findings, this erogenous zone swelled when stimulated and "swells out greatly at the end of orgasm."

In the 1970s, while treating women suffering from urinary stress incontinence (USI), John D. Perry, Ph.D., and Beverly Whipple, R.N., Ph.D., made an important discovery that led them to the G-spot. Typically, women suffering from USI have weak or atrophied pelvic muscles. The strength of these muscles can be measured through biofeedback and can be strengthened by teaching women Kegel exercises (a technique for strengthening the pubococcygeus or PC muscle). However, Perry and Whipple discovered that some of the women who supposedly suffered from USI had very strong pelvic muscles. Furthermore, these same women with strong pelvic muscles often stated that the only time they (accidentally) lost fluid through their urethra was during intercourse.

Much like Columbus's epic journey, setting forth for the Indies and discovering America instead, Dr. Perry and Dr. Whipple discovered their own land of milk and honey, which they aptly named "the Gräfenberg spot" in honor of Dr. Ernst Gräfenberg's early research.

At the 1980 national meeting of the American Association of Sex Educators, Counselors and Therapists, and the 1980 international meeting of the Society for the Scientific Study of Sex, Perry and Whipple presented their findings about the G-spot and female ejaculation. Later, in 1982, along with Alice Kahn Ladas, they published a book explaining the Gräfenberg spot, female ejaculation, the importance of healthy pelvic muscles, and new understandings of the human orgasm. This book, popular for many years, is titled *The G Spot and Other Discoveries About Human Sexuality* and is still in print as of this writing, with an updated edition published in 2005.

Since the release of *The G Spot and Other Discoveries About Human Sexuality*, more has been learned about the G-spot and female ejaculation. As each new doorway to knowledge is unlocked and opened, we find yet another doorway waiting. The more we learn, the more mysteries await us. History unfolds while no one is watching.

2

The Technique

Now that you know a little about the G-spot, you're probably wondering how you can test the G-spot technique firsthand.

Let me commend you if you've read this far and haven't skipped ahead. One of the most frequent complaints women voice about poor lovers is having partners with a "vaginal objective." These "vaginal marksmen" wants to kiss once or twice, perhaps fondle the breasts, and then move right to the clitoris or vagina. If you've taken the time to read this far, you're likely not a vaginal marksman. (They are either thumbing through the book, looking for pictures, or have skipped right to Step 10 and will have to back up, reread, and likely will never get this straight. A year from now they'll be the ones responsible for rumors that the G-spot doesn't exist). You, on the other hand, will find the truth, since you have displayed the two most important attributes to success in helping your lover achieve a G-spot orgasm: patience and self-control.

As a side note, one critical reviewer of the 2001 edition of this book praised it for being to the point and written in simple terms, but believed the author assumed that all men were poor lovers. I can see how this reviewer drew that conclusion. I feel I should emphasize that not all men are poor lovers. I applaud you, and believe you will be successful in your quest.

On the other hand, if the G-spot orgasm were something easy to achieve, nearly every woman on the planet would know what it is and how to do it. Right? Most would have found this spot (as they find their clitoris, during exploratory masturbation), and would be enjoying its pleasures. But as we know, nothing could be further from the truth. Even today, the G-spot remains arcane, obscure, misunderstood, and a topic of curiosity.

As evidence of this, look at the Internet educational service called KISISS (Kinsey Institute Sexuality Information Service for Students). KISISS allows Indiana University students to ask questions about sex in an anonymous fashion. After each question is answered, both the question and answer are posted for other site users to read. Interestingly enough, at the time of the first writing of this book, the number one most frequently read question was: "What is the G-spot and where can I find it?"[26] The sheer fact that college university students (and visitors) read this question more than any other question lends us insight. Clearly, it shows that even today the G-spot is still a mystery.

Like ships passing in the night, people repeatedly overlook the G-spot. As many women pass through their sexual lives, they mature, explore their own bodies, masturbate, have intercourse, bear children, and often never find their own G-spot. Similarly, the partners who share in their lovemaking also overlook this special spot.

Until two decades ago, even many of the doctors who examine women daily—gynecologists and obstetricians—were unsure of the G-spot's existence. In defense of these physicians, we should remember that (1) the G-spot cannot be seen without dissection of the anterior vagina wall and (2) it is virtually unnoticeable until stimulated. Since gynecologists and obstetricians are not in the practice of stimulating their patients, it stands to reason they would fail to notice the spot.

With all this in mind, if you truly want to find the elusive G-spot and help your partner feel *absolutely the best* orgasm she's ever felt—a spasming, screaming-and-thrashing-in-ecstasy G-spot orgasm—patience and self-control are nearly mandatory. If you follow the ten-step technique, once you learn and become familiar with the G-spot orgasm, you'll be able to condense the technique and efficiently help your lover produce results much of the time. But like any worthwhile endeavor, the technique takes practice. The more you do it, the more quickly you'll learn to identify certain body signs that allow you to move on to the next step.

The same is true of your partner. If you have a steady sex partner, after she loses her "G-spot virginity" she will also learn to read her body signs and will be able to hit the G-spot climax sooner, and in a wide variety of positions.

Step 1: Priming

Although it's possible to help a woman achieve a G-spot orgasm on the first sexual encounter, the surest bet is with steady partners who are familiar and comfortable together.

This is because of preexisting emotional bonds and qualities. In order to fully let go, many women need to feel safe, loved, relaxed, and secure with their partners' sexual prowess and understanding.

Recommendation number one: As I said earlier, it's wise not to mention the G-spot orgasm to your partner in advance. If you tell her you want to "try something new" you'll be fostering expectations in her that may be counterproductive when you actually get down to lovemaking. She'll feel the need to "perform" without understanding the details. Therefore, she will be apprehensive and edgy when it's helpful to be exactly the opposite: relaxed and comfortable.

> "It's critical that foreplay start long before you reach the bedroom."
> —Anonymous

I really can't stress enough the value of her being relaxed. Instead of telling your lover about your covert plan, set up the opportunity to "show" her. Sit down with your lover and tell her that you'd love to take her out for dinner and a show, then return home and spend the evening making slow, passionate love. Be sure to mention the second part of this plan so your lover doesn't get the wrong impression—that the two of you are going to spend the entire evening out together. This will do two things for you. One, your lover will appreciate your candor and the romance of the gesture; two, it will prime her for lovemaking. If your relationship is fair or better, she'll probably be thinking about the lovemaking long before you order dinner or choose a movie.

Beyond this preparation, be sure to groom your fingers prior to your date. Because much of this technique involves stimulation of the delicate vaginal tissues, be sure your fingernails are short, clean, and smooth to avoid damaging the soft tissues of her body. Wear your favorite cologne. Look and feel your best.

Step 2: Foreplay

When you go out for your big evening, as you wine and dine her, *talk to her*. In *The 10-Second Kiss*, a book filled with wise and sound advice for rekindling the spark in any fading relationship, author Ellen Kreidman discusses the value of compliments, kissing, hugs, and laughter, as well as the importance of heart-to-heart communication. "A relationship is only as deep as its level of communication,"[27] the author states. And this is indeed true. Couples who are open, can share their feelings, and feel secure with each other are primed for success with the G-spot orgasm.

If you're a new couple, carrying on a conversation over dinner should be easy, since we're always eager to learn more about a new partner. What type of childhood did she have? What's her favorite color? Who is her favorite relative, and why? Who is her least favorite, and why? What type of music does she like? Who is her favorite celebrity?

For those of you in longer relationships, you probably already know what music she listens to, her favorite color, and her favorite relatives (and your least favorite of her relatives). Because of this, all too often it's easy to get caught up in surface talk—recapping the day, or reiterating problems you handled, what bills you paid, whether the lawn got mowed, etc. The key to moving from surface chit-chat to deeper and more meaningful conversation is to ask questions that evoke thought, opinion, and feelings; preferably questions which steer the conversation away from the more mundane aspects of day-to-day life. Search for questions that are positive, that tap her dreams, and that are fun and thought provoking. For example:

If she won an all-expense-paid vacation to any destination in the world, where would she go, and why would she choose that destination?

If she became a castaway on a tropical island, what would she do? Would she enjoy it or hate it?

What was the best advice her parents ever gave her? What was the worst?

What was the last thing she did that she's thankful she choose to do?

What is her first memory?

If she had a million dollars to give away, whom would she give it to? A struggling family? A charity? A pet shelter? Why?

Have fun with this. Be creative.

And as you talk to her, don't forget to touch her. Hold hands. Touch her gently on the shoulder or arm. Brush the hair from her face. Studies have shown that the hormone oxytocin, often referred to as the "touch hormone," is released in our bodies whenever we are touched. In addition, as author Darcy Cole puts it in her book *Seduce Me! How to Ignite Your Partner's Passion* (recommended), "Oxytocin creates in us a sense of attachment to the person who is touching us. It also creates in us a desire to be touched even more."[28]

Beyond casual touching and talking, remember to compliment her. There are few better ways to encourage conversation than compliments or light humor.

Step 3: More Foreplay

After you've taken her out for an enchanting evening and have returned home, continue the foreplay. If you haven't already given her flowers, this might be the perfect time to do so. Talk over coffee. Slow dance in the living room. Give her the "full meal" treatment.

Remind her of how beautiful she is and how much you enjoy being with her. Boost the intimacy. Continue to talk to her, possibly giving her a light massage to help her further relax. Most likely, with a few more kisses, some light petting, and additional compliments, the two of you will be stripping each other as if your clothes are on fire—falling into bed together as if it were the only pool of water in the world. And this is when you need to gently take control. If this is your steady partner and you've primed her the week before your date, she'll likely be wet and ready to fall into your standard lovemaking. Seize control by telling her you want to take it slow this time. Remind her that you want to make slow love to her—that you want to spend some time pleasing and savoring *her* and making *her* feel loved. Many women are natural caregivers, which makes it challenging for them to simply relax and assume the reverse role. If this is the case with your partner, validate the fact that she's always caring for others, and now it's her turn to be pampered. She'll love you for that.

Ask her to lie back and make herself comfortable, and remind her that you love her. If she has beautiful breasts, tell her so. If it's her eyes, her long legs, or her full sensual lips that you like, tell her so. Praise is a key element within any relationship. It costs nothing to give but can be priceless when received. It helps us maintain a healthy self-image and self-worth while making us feel respected, desirable, and loved. If you love your partner, praise her. Tell her what you love about her; not just her physical beauties, but her emotional qualities, her skills, her wit, whatever it is you truly admire.

By doing this, you're promoting a deep sense of intimacy and comfort while keeping her aroused. Kiss her. Nibble on her lips. Kiss her throat, the lobes of her ears, her eyelids— all of them can be erotic and arousing spots.

For most women, by the time you've spent a few minutes kissing all about her face, nibbling the lips, kissing the eyelids, perhaps blowing in her ear, and dragging your lips over her neck and down to her shoulders, you'll probably notice her beginning to inch upward or pressing your face toward her breasts and arching her back. If she's a bit forward or bold, she may seek you out with her hand or guide your hand to her breast. She may even tell you she wants you—but don't sell off the million-dollar orgasm that cheaply. A critical element here is keeping all your attention, physical and emotional, focused at breast level or above.

Step 4: Teasing

So here you are, in bed together, possibly naked or half-naked by this point, very aroused and ready. You've (both) been thinking about this moment ever since you first mentioned the evening out. This is the part where your patience and self-control are beginning to come into play, and she may look so inviting that it's tough to pass up her offer to take you now. But don't sell yourself short.

Lavish her with kisses. If she enjoys having her neck kissed, by all means oblige. If she enjoys breast stimulation, nuzzle and fondle and tease her breasts. At this point, you can bend the rule of focusing all attention at the breast level (and above) by rubbing her stomach. This is an important step in the arousal process. The purpose is to increase blood flow in the pelvic area. Work your hand back and forth across her stomach and down her abdomen very slowly. You don't want her to think you're targeting the vulva, so move slowly and randomly until you've reached the area just above the pubic hairline. As part of the tease, don't drop your hand any lower, even if she tries to move it there or tells you she wants you and starts pulling you toward her.

The reason you don't want to touch any lower than the abdomen (yet) is because it breaks the bond you're working to build. Some women have experienced the vagina marksman and may be emotionally turned off when your interest is transferred to the vagina (if it happens too soon). When this occurs, it often signifies the end of the bonding process and the beginning of sex. This switch can be flicked as easily as a light switch. And when it happens, the mist of enchantment lifts.

Continue to nuzzle her breasts, kiss her, nibble at her neck, or whatever shows your love. Your goal is to continue increasing the emotional bond between you, and she will unconsciously give you signs as the strength of the bond deepens. Remember, you're about to provide the stimulus for an orgasm that is unlike anything she's ever felt. In order to reach it, she'll be slowly transferring her trust to you. She'll need to feel cherished, safe, and adored in order to do so without holding back.

> *"The clitoris can really distract a woman. Stay away from it the first few times you use the technique. You'll have time for it later."* —R. B.

As you continue nuzzling, kissing, nibbling in whatever way turns her on, you are watching for two "go ahead" signs before moving to Step 5. The first sign is the most important. You must continue stimulation until she is virtually smashing your head into her chest, breathing heavily, tugging at you as if she's trying to pull you inside her. Once you become aware of this, start watching (or sensing) for the second sign: movements in her hips. The hips never lie, and you want her thrusting them upward. If she's not thrusting, arching, or twisting her hips, she's not ready. So continue nuzzling and sucking at her breasts or otherwise stimulating her until her hips move. If need be, move your hand a little lower on her abdomen to brush the upper edge of the pubic hair as you rub. Before long, both of these signs will appear.

Step 5: The "Go Ahead" Sign

Once you have the two "go ahead" signs of arching hips and tugging, absolutely don't break contact with her breasts, chest, or face. Keep your head and face at chest level or above. This sends the unspoken message *I'm still with you*—and that you're not merely moving on to focus on her vagina.

With the hand you've been using to massage her abdomen, slowly trace down to rub her upper and inner thighs—again, without touching the vagina and setting off the vagina marksman alarm. If you like, reach around and squeeze the lower half of either buttock in a teasing way. Massage the muscles gently. Working the flesh actually tugs at the edge of the vulva, helping to open the labia and helping her become more ready and wanton. This massage also increases blood flow in the pelvis, arousing and heightening sensitivity.

Trace your fingers up and down her thighs, provocatively circling her "magic triangle." Brushing the edges will ensure that her hips continue to thrust. Above all, remember to focus on her face to hold the emotional bond you've established.

Step 6: Hovering

By now, she should be thrusting her hips wantonly and moving in a way to actually encourage you to touch her vagina. If she's bold, she may try to massage herself or try to guide your hand (or your penis) to the area. Don't let her. If necessary, remind her lovingly that you want to spend more time just touching and savoring her. If she wants to massage herself, encourage her to massage her breasts. Moreover, encourage her simply to just lie back and enjoy it.

Your next step is to move your hand above her womanhood and hover it there, just brushing the tips of the pubic hair. (If she's clean-shaven or waxed, she'll still sense your hand there.) If she's already really aroused, this will drive her absolutely crazy. She'll sense your hand and the heat it gives off and may impulsively arch her hips toward it. Expect this reaction and raise your hand to avoid contact.

While hovering, you may even tug at the hair lightly. You need not tease her in this way for more than two or three minutes, but be sure to allow your hand to hover above her womanhood long enough for her to show some type of acknowledgment—even if it's only a moan.

Many women harbor inhibitions about being verbal or displaying their sexual needs or desire. The underlying significance of the hovering is twofold. Not only does it increase your lover's arousal, but it also encourages her to react and helps to break through any inhibitions she may be struggling with. It should be abundantly clear that you are deliberately (almost mercilessly) teasing her, searching for a reaction, and this gives her a justifiable reason to react without compromising her ego or sacrificing dignity. You've compelled, almost forced, her to react. And for many women, once they have reacted the first time and break the barrier, it's easier and acceptable to react again.

After you've hovered and obtained a reaction, allow your fingers to trace up and down the flesh on either side of her vagina. By "flesh" I don't mean the labia or lips, but rather the mounds on either side of the vulva. Touch them very lightly. This is an extension of the tease and should further fuel the fires of arousal.

Continue this for a while and slowly transition from featherlight touches to a soft massage. Few people realize there are muscles on either side of the vaginal opening, so take a little time to gently massage these muscles, relaxing them.

"Before we learned your technique, I had seriously considered having my breasts augmented because my husband tended to ignore them. I think that reading your book helped him grasp the importance of kissing and fondling my breasts. Whether a woman's breasts are small or large, it's usually very pleasurable having them nuzzled and played with. I know several women who feel this way. Stimulating the breasts is an important part of lovemaking for me. Thanks for emphasizing this in your book." —C. S.

After you've massaged these muscles for a moment, trace her vagina with your fingers, using a finger on either side of her vagina to lightly pull back and spread open the labia. The labia are a very sensitive and erogenous area, yet many women report they are overlooked during lovemaking. So spend a little time here, flattening the genital lips and tracing them with your fingertips. Gently tug at them and spread them open. This sense of the vagina being opened will often trigger a high vaginal craving, and she'll want that void filled.

If you like, you may even stroke the clitoris lightly—but don't linger there, as the clitoris can be very distractive to firsttime G-spot orgasms. If you've thought of the clitoris as the primary stimulus point for a woman, you'll want to retrain your thinking. From this point on, think of the G-spot as the main stimulation and the clitoris as a "booster" or secondary stimulus. Remember that the women polled report that G-spot orgasms are significantly more intense than clitoral orgasms, both in duration and fulfillment.

As discussed earlier, blended orgasms are an exception to this rule and will certainly warrant future exploration. But for tonight, this special first night, avoid the clitoris unless she really needs an extra boost.

In some ways, the G-spot and the clitoris are like internal/external counterparts. G-spot virgins, who have spent a lifetime thinking of their clitoris as their primary stimulation, may get so involved trying to give themselves a clitoral orgasm that they lose track of the G-spot stimulation you're trying to build. While it has not been scientifically proven, our belief is that "single-taskers" can only focus on one form of internal stimulation at a time, just as they can only focus on one form of external stimulus at a time. It follows that multitaskers are more likely to succeed at blended orgasms. Whether or not this is the case, I advise you try to keep your lover away from her clitoris for this night. Touch it enough to tease, and then move on.

Bear in mind, through this whole process: Never break contact with her body from the breasts up. Return frequently to kiss her lips, and ward off her advances if she tries to pull you onto her.

Step 7: Locating Her G-Spot

By now, there should be no doubt she's ready. She should be moaning (at least quietly), thrashing her hips, arching her back, and urging you on. And as you finally dip your finger into that moist warm wetness, your patience and self-control will be tested to the maximum. But don't give up—you're almost there!

Slide your finger into her very slowly, dipping in very shallowly at first to allow your finger to become moist, pulling out and dipping in again. As you do this, dip a little deeper each time, keeping light pressure on the front wall of the vagina—all the while being careful not to scratch those sensitive folds of velvet.

When touching a woman, many lovers make the error of plunging a finger as deeply into the vagina as possible and wiggling it around, not realizing that, aside from the hidden G-spot, most of the sensitive nerves lie within the first 2 inches of the vagina. Hence the adage: It's not what you've got, but how you use it. So don't make the error of plunging. Your goal here is to tantalize the outer nerve endings while allowing your finger to become sufficiently lubricated to visit the hidden depths.

If your partner is not well lubricated, you may want to use a suitable lubricant. Her being "dry" does not mean she is not aroused. Diet, hormonal levels, medications, and menstrual cycle can all affect vaginal lubrication. Wetness is not a valid gauge of arousal.

Finally, slide your index finger into her, skimming the front or upper wall of the vagina. This is the critical process of locating the G-spot. As you continue to kiss her, teasing her nipples or sucking her breasts, concentrate for a moment on what your finger encounters.

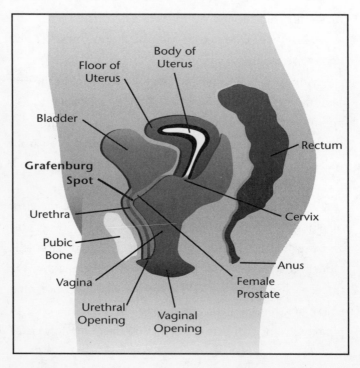

Study the diagram on page 50. This may help you better understand the location of the G-spot when the time comes.

In most women, about 1 to 1.5 inches inside, you'll feel a slightly textured area of skin. (It feels somewhat like the roof of your mouth.) This textured area is the Skene's glands. Immediately beyond this textured area lies the pelvic bone, which is often hard to feel. The G-spot is hidden in what feels like a "valley" just beyond the pelvic bone. If you go too far and pass the G-spot, you'll feel a smooth "plateau" that is flat for an inch or two, then curves inward toward the opening of the cervix. (Although it is hard to reach, the opening of the cervix is also a very erotic spot if caressed lightly.) If you go too far and reach this plateau, back up just past the bottom of the "valley" and rub the downslope between the valley and the edge of the textured area.

In most cases, the G-spot feels like a small bean or a very small nipple felt through the wall of the vagina. With some women, it can't be perceived at all (which helps explain why it has been so difficult to find). Just as with breasts or nipples, some women have small G-spots and others have larger ones. (Postmenopausal women, especially, have small G-spots.) I've heard reports of G-spots having the diameter of a quarter, but the average is probably closer to the size of a pinto bean.

Once you've found the G-spot—or are in the vicinity of where it should be, if you can't actually feel it—begin rubbing very lightly in a circular manner, as if you were tracing the rim of a quarter, at the rate of about one revolution per second. The pressure you apply at first should be about the same as you would use to write your name on a steam-fogged mirror. You can use one finger, or two, whichever feels more comfortable to you and best matches the size of your partner.

Step 8: Stimulating the G-Spot

Okay, you're finally there, rubbing the G-spot. So why isn't anything happening?

When you first touch the G-spot, don't be surprised if you don't get an immediate reaction. Just continue rubbing between the bottom of the valley and the innermost edge of the textured area.

In most cases, women will make comments such as "That feels good" or "Stay right there" or "That feels so different." But if you don't get any response at all, don't panic. Think of the G-spot as being similar to the nipple. When you first touch a nipple it is soft and only relatively sensitive. But as blood flows to the area and the nipple grows erect and aroused,

> *"Keep a fresh towel and lots of lubrication in the bedroom."* —D. T.

the sensitivity increases in a dramatic flourish. The G-spot is much the same. As you begin to caress it in a slow, circular manner, you will soon feel the area swell. It may become more porous and have an almost grainy feel. And it will most definitely become very sensitive.

If the G-spot is massaged without prior arousal, many women find it uncomfortable. This is one of the key reasons that some people fail to find the G-spot. Halfhearted pioneers often search for any spot that gives a woman greater pleasure. Yet if these seekers blindly happen upon the G-spot (without proper arousal) the woman may report minor discomfort or an "uncomfortable feeling," steering them away. This is an important point to remember. If you try to move through the G-spot technique faster in the future and skip over steps, the G-spot may not be properly aroused when you reach it. Always follow the steps and watch for the "go ahead" signs from your partner as you move from one step to the next.

Rhythm is the absolute key here. As long as you maintain a steady rhythm, slow-building waves of ecstasy begin to wash in. Each wave that comes will be a little higher in intensity than the previous, and they will begin to cascade and surge faster and faster, until a point when just as one wave is beginning to fade, the next is already swelling.

When a women tries to stimulate her own G-spot, she may be inclined to stroke the area faster and firmer as the waves grow more intense, trying to push the wave to crest and break over into the ecstasy she senses just beyond. The problem is, she can overstimulate the G-spot and inhibit the orgasm. This is critical to remember when your lover begs you to stroke faster or firmer. Be cautious about giving in. Maintain a slow, even rhythm at first.

On the other hand, if you've been stimulating her G-spot for ten minutes (or longer) at one revolution per second and she can't "crest over," it may be time to try a different touch. Remember that all women are different. Some women need a slightly firmer touch. For some, a side-to-side or up-and-down finger movement is more effective than a circular one. Some women prefer stimulation with one finger while others prefer two or more. For yet others, slight variations in the speed are more effective— or a combination of any of these techniques. This is where practice, judgment, and experimentation will come into play. I recommend at first using the light, circular, one-revolution-per-second method. Our research has shown that it is the most effective.

> "The great thing about the G-spot is you can do it nearly anywhere. On our first 'date night,' I was really eager and started fingering my wife and massaging her G-spot during the movie. She was moaning quietly and orgasmed within five minutes. It was exciting for both of us because we were doing it in public." —Anonymous

In many instances when lovers were urged to move faster or firmer, and they complied, the orgasm faded instead of growing. When the original slow and light touch was resumed, success soon followed.

The good news is that there appears to be a "point of no return" with G-spot orgasms. After her first experience, your lover will likely convey this to you ardently. While it may take fifteen or more minutes of stimulation —a great workout for your forearm—most women reach a point where waves of pleasure are building and cascading so rapidly the orgasm becomes nearly inevitable.

When one woman was asked if she could "will," or stop, a clitoral or vaginal orgasm from occurring, she replied, "Why, yes. Certainly." But in discussing her G-spot experience, the same woman stated, "I reached a point where I couldn't stop it from coming, even if I wanted to!"

When you finally get to witness your lover thrashing and screaming in the throes of pure ecstasy, it's very difficult not to become excited yourself and begin rubbing at the G-spot with great enthusiasm. When some lovers see their partner in such ecstasy—especially if she has her first (visible) ejaculation, they often experience orgasm themselves. However, if you can maintain control and keep up the G-spot stimulation, her orgasm may continue for minutes on end. This is how some couples state they can maintain an orgasm for 20 or more minutes! One couple even reported an orgasm that lasted 40 minutes and only stopped because neither partner could stand any more.

Step 9: The "Big O" Draws Near

In most cases, aside from the initial slight swelling of the G-spot, you won't notice any changes inside the vagina. When dealing with women who are new to the G-spot orgasm, you'll often find the muscles in your forearm begin to burn before you feel the first vaginal contraction squeezing against your finger. Most of our survey respondents state that 20 minutes of G-spot stimulation was required the first time. It will likely go faster in the future. So, again, it's time to use that patience and self-control. You haven't come this far only to stop now. And if you do stop now, you'll likely disappoint your lover, who is aware of this massive ecstasy burgeoning inside her.

As the G-spot orgasm grows near—the Big O—the first thing you'll notice is a constricting of the vagina that begins with one of the waves. With the next wave the vagina will constrict again, relax, then quickly return with the next wave, building and building to a point where the vagina is so constantly constricted the muscles begin to spasm and quiver. Sometimes the constriction is so tight it will eject your finger! About the same time you notice the first constriction, you'll also likely notice a greater wetness. In fact, some women become very wet, to the point the suction of the finger causes slurping noises and a clear fluid actually begins to weep from the vagina. As discussed earlier, this is the wonder of female ejaculation. Rather than necessarily always squirting, it often weeps out of the urethral opening and into the vagina.

> *"For a real treat, try having her lie on her back on a table or counter. Have her bottom positioned near the edge. If you squat in front of her, you can hold her labia open and watch as she orgasms and ejaculates. It's amazing to see the juice flow down your hand as her vagina contracts and sucks on your finger."* —I. W.

If this occurs, you may notice that the consistency of this fluid differs from the normal milky lubricant produced by the vagina in that it's more watery and less slick. Your finger may lose its slickness, and since the area is so sensitive, you may want to pause and quickly apply an approved sexual lubricant. Have some lubricant available before things get started. As a general rule, the slicker your finger stays, the better.

Step 10: You're There!

You're there! As the wetness increases, the vagina will begin to convulse violently. As mentioned, some women constrict so hard it forces the finger out of the vagina. By this time, your lover will undoubtedly be thrashing wildly and screaming, "Don't stop! Don't stop! Oh, God, don't stop!" or "Faster! Faster! Faster!" But regardless of how frantic your lover becomes, regardless of how excited you get by watching her ecstasy, try to control your motions.

As she finally crests over the top, if she is like most women, she will scream. This scream differs from the usual scream of orgasm—more of a guttural expelling sound than a gasping sound. Picture a woman giving birth, her head hunched forward, her fists clenching her knees, and imagine the sound she might make—you're on the right track. Now, at the moment your partner cries out, she may ejaculate, if she hasn't already done so. This is especially true of G-spot virgins. While it defies the findings of scientific research, many of our respondents describe their first G-spot orgasm as the wettest—almost as if the fluid has been locked up for years and you're opening the dam, setting it free.

One theory is that many of these couples simply don't "work" as hard on subsequent sessions as they did during their first G-spot experience. The degree of emotional bonding and the duration of stimulation may also play a role in determining the volume of fluid produced and the intensity of the orgasm. While these topics are worthy of future exploration, they need not detain us here. At this point, simply keep your finger moving until your lover asks you to stop or the orgasm fades. Typically, she will ride that wave for one or two full minutes, then the orgasm will lessen, and the area will become too sensitive for you to touch for a couple of minutes.

When you witness your partner experience such an orgasm, you will be completely rewarded for all your "work." Just watching her writhe and knowing the intense pleasure you are helping to provide is a great reward in itself.

Most men will want to join her as they sense this wave fading. The change from a finger to a swollen penis may delight her, and by this point, having watched her thrash and scream, feeling the warm wetness on your finger and hand, your self-control will likely be gone. So as long as she's willing, jump in and enjoy the orgasm with her. Feeling a wet, contracting vagina sucking at the penis can be an experience neither of you will forget! You'll want it again and again, and common quickies simply won't have the same appeal anymore.

3

Afterward

The Little Death

Immediately after the orgasm, a few women pass through a phase called "the little death." This phase is a five-to-ten-second period in which the woman may appear to faint or seems to stop breathing. If this occurs, don't panic. Women who have passed through the little death frequently state that they were so overwhelmed with pleasure they "floated in delirium" for a brief period. Other women may have a tendency to pant briefly before or during the orgasm, resulting in either hyperventilation or hypoventilation. In either case, a combination of the tremendous release of stress, sudden slowing of the heart, and a redirection of oxygen-rich (or suddenly depleted) blood cells can bring about the little death.

After five or ten seconds, your lover should dreamily open her eyes. When you ask if she's okay—and you should—she'll likely tell you everything is fine, that she was simply enjoying the moment.

If your partner does actually faint and remains unresponsive for more than 15 or 20 seconds, you may have a medical emergency on your hands and should contact medical assistance immediately. Again, as a responsible party, it is your duty to know your partner's health status before engaging in sexual activity.

Sharing the Experience

In one survey, we asked women to express how they felt after their G-spot experience. Women responding to this survey were instructed to indicate their feelings by either writing in a comment or making multiple-choice selections.

Of these respondents, an overwhelming 97 percent indicated feeling "joyous/elated" after their first G-spot experience. Other leading answers were: "loving/romantic" (89 percent), "thankful" (84 percent), and "satiated/fulfilled" (82 percent).

While the vast majority of responses and comments were favorable, 47 percent also indicated feeling "embarrassment" or "curiosity" intermixed with other feelings. A few (3 percent) said their feelings of embarrassment stemmed from becoming too "verbal" or "expressive" during the sexual episode. A much larger group stated that their embarrassment arose from fear they had "wet the bed" or "lost bladder control" during the intense orgasm.

In some of these cases, women stated that they had no idea females could ejaculate and therefore concluded they had "wet the bed." One telltale comment we frequently received was this:

> *"I knew other women could ejaculate, but I didn't know I could."*

As conscientious partners, it's important to be aware of this information. If your lover ejaculates during G-spot stimulation, she may fear she has "wet the bed" and may hide or avoid discussing her "problem" due to personal embarrassment. Undoubtedly, she will feel bad about herself and equally bad about what's happened, even if the experience brought her great pleasure.

To thwart these hidden tensions and keep them from reemerging in the future, be sure to talk openly with your partner about your first mutual G-spot adventure. Discuss the phenomenon of female ejaculation. Learn how she feels about it: what she knows, or doesn't know. Reassure her that female ejaculations are physiologically normal. Reaffirm that they are natural and shouldn't be a source of embarrassment. Be open and honest. If you enjoyed it, tell her so. If it excited you, tell her so. If you're ready to go again, tell her so. Promote sexual expression. Explore. Try new positions. Be creative. Make it fun and loving.

Above all, make it good for both of you.

4

G-Spot-friendly Coitus

Take a moment and congratulate yourself again. Thanks to the knowledge you've gained through your investment in this book, you'll find yourself being constantly aware of the G-spot during all phases of foreplay and lovemaking. And because of this awareness, you and your partner will quickly learn to adjust and angle yourselves to promote G-spot stimulation and derive greater pleasure during normal intercourse—something you never would have imagined prior to reading this book.

"How can a man derive more pleasure due to the G-spot?" you might ask.

If you're male and you've witnessed a G-spot orgasm, the answer is obvious. For most men, the thought of having their penis inside a wet, spasming, tightly contracting vagina during G-spot orgasm has unlimited appeal. And as you and your partner grow more familiar with the G-spot, you may soon be able to cultivate G-spot orgasms using the penis.

As an added benefit, as your partner grows more familiar and comfortable with G-spot orgasms, she'll be able to attain them with greater speed, more reliability, and in a variety of coital positions, thus including the G-spot in other realms of lovemaking, forging ahead toward blended orgasms.

"So where should we start?" you might ask.

As I'll cover in chapter 5, Exploring Other Possibilities, a variety of sex toys are available for stimulating the G-spot. Most of these toys can be used with a partner as well as solo. Beyond the joys these toys offer, couples can also experiment with G-spot-friendly coital positions.

"What are G-spot-friendly coital positions?"

These are sexual positions that promote contact between the G-spot and the penis. While there are a va-

> *"My wife and I like to lie on our sides in a 69 position. I can perform cunnilingus and massage her G-spot while she gives me head or massages me with lotion. It drives us both crazy."* —R. G.

riety of G-spot-friendly positions, the favored one is commonly referred to as the "woman on top" position.

Woman on Top

In this position, the man lies on his back with legs slightly parted and extended flat. The woman then straddles him, facing forward. This position is favorable because it is face to face and allows expression, kissing, nuzzling, and stimulation of the breasts during intercourse. It also allows the woman to angle her hips so the penis contacts her G-spot. By leaning forward or backward, the woman can adjust the pressure of the penis against the G-spot.

Missionary with Pillow

A second G-spot-friendly position is a variation of the missionary position. By placing a thick pillow (or two pillows) beneath the woman's buttocks (so she's lying with her head downhill), the man will be able to bring his penis in contact with the G-spot.

Missionary with Footstool

As a variation of the Missionary with Pillow position, you can use a short padded footstool (with sturdy legs) in place of the pillow. Since this position is more radical than the version with the pillow, you should try it out on the floor first.

To begin, the woman lies flat on her back and raises her hips so that the footstool can be slid beneath her buttocks (a pillow under her back and head is often desirable to provide cushion or avoid rugburns). The man then kneels to crouch over her in a push-up position. Because of the firmness of both the floor and the footstool, the contact between the man and the woman is felt more solidly, with the man having nearly all control of the pace and thrusting.

If your footstool is equipped with either a square base or blunt "feet" that won't damage or impale your mattress, this position can also be attained on a bed. Using the footstool on the bed provides new and unique sensations—the mattress pro-

> *"If you want a thrill, have her lie on her back. Lie on your side facing her. Have her throw her nearest leg over the top your legs so you can rub her G-spot and slide your [penis] inside her at the same time. That way, your finger is massaging her G-spot and your [penis]! When she starts contracting, it will drive you both crazy."*
> —D. J.

vides cushion and allows the woman to "rock" in addition to the man's thrusting.

Kneeling Missionary

G-spot/penis contact also occurs in a variation of the missionary position. With both partners on the bed, the man kneels or sits on folded knees, keeping his body upright or nearly upright.

Legs-Up Missionary

In another variation of missionary, the woman lies flat on her back with her legs lifted upright. The man can then place her calves or ankles on his shoulders as he enters her.

Rear Entry with Pillow

For more direct stimulation of the G-spot, try a rear-entry approach, again using pillows to lift the woman's pelvis. In this position, the woman lies on her stomach and slides a pillow under the lower half of her pelvis, thus lifting her rear. She spreads her legs slightly, and the man kneels over her and enters her from behind.

Standing Doggy Style

Another great G-spot friendly position is "doggy style." If the man stands and the woman bends at the waist at a partial angle (for example, leaning forward with the hands braced against a wall), the underside of the penis will contact the G-spot. For couples who are similar in height and enjoy sex in the shower, this can be a fun position. However, the angle depends greatly on the man's penis. While some penises stand straight out during erection (at a 90-degree angle to the body), others tend to stand more upright, with the penis head near the abdomen. In the latter case, the woman must stand nearly erect (or the man must lean forward) for G-spot contact to be made.

Kneeling Doggy Style

Doggy style can also be performed with the woman on her hands and knees and the man kneeling behind her.

Furniture Fun

Various pieces of furniture can add dimensions to your lovemaking. For example, it doesn't take much imagination to see the possibilities of a rocking chair. Try having her face the chair and kneel on it while he enters from behind. Or have him sit in the chair, while she drapes her legs over the arms of the chair and sits in his lap; she can choose to either face him or away.

A flat surface such as a table is another common option. The woman lies back with her legs in the air; the man holds her feet together while penetrating her.

An ottoman can be another lovemaking platform, as can a wingback chair, or a porch swing.

Beyond these, there are numerous other positions that are G-spot friendly. One couple reported that their favorite position is with the woman sitting atop the washing machine while the man stands facing her. During the spin cycle, the machine causes her G-spot and vagina to vibrate against his penis, bringing both of them great pleasure and *multiple* climaxes. They also stated that if she faces the washer and leans forward, the machine vibrates against her clitoris while he enters her from behind.

Another couple said they enjoy using a thin G-spot vibrator with ample lubrication. As the woman nears climax, she withdraws the vibrator and moves it to her clitoris as her spouse enters her, allowing them to climax together.

Endless possibilities abound as you and your partner explore together. As you sample each pleasure, remember also to savor what you feel along the way. Take time and make it fun. Rather than racing to the destination, take some time and enjoy the journey.

5

Exploring Other Possibilities

Toys

In today's market, there are many sex toys designed to stimulate the G-spot. Among these are vibrating eggs, weighted balls, vibrators, and specially curved vibrators designed to reach the G-spot.

Vibrating Eggs

Vibrating eggs—sometimes referred to as "bullets"—typically consist of an egg that may be inserted into the vagina (or rolled over the body), and a short cord that leads to a remote control for turning it on and adjusting the vibration speed. A variety of these devices are available, ranging from low-end models with a simple on/off switch to dual-speed models (high/low), five- and six-speed models, and even high-end models that include a computer chip to randomize the vibration speed and intensity. Vibrating eggs serve as an excellent arousal tool and can be used by couples during foreplay or for solo enjoyment. They can also be held easily in the hand during intercourse for rubbing a partner's breasts or other erogenous areas.

Weighted Balls

Weighted balls, often called Ben Wa balls, may also be rolled over the body as a source of foreplay, but they are usually inserted inside the vagina prior to lovemaking. According to reports we've received, many women use these balls to spark arousal or for their own self-pleasure. Some state that they wear them around the house, when they jog, when they go on dates, or even to the office, and are more likely to wear them when they feel confident they'll be "getting lucky." Weighted balls also serve as an excellent personal arousal tool. One disadvantage is that they can be difficult to remove and are often made of (cold) metal. A variation, called "Smart Balls," has a string or plastic cord for easier removal.

> "Sometimes the muscles in my forearm cramp up while I'm rubbing her G-spot. I've found that keeping a G-spot vibrator next to the bed is a good idea in case my hand cramps. The secret is to buy a thin one. Some of the vibrators available are so big that when she starts contracting they become uncomfortable." —K. R.

G-Spot Vibrators

Much like vibrating eggs, G-spot vibrators come in a wide array of sizes, with a similar variety of vibration speeds. The shaft of a typical G-spot vibrator is straight, with the final inch or so of the tip angled at 30 to 40 degrees.

As a general rule, when starting out with a G-spot vibrator, smaller is better. A smaller shaft allows more flexibility, so the tip can be guided more easily to the G-spot.

> *"My girlfriend and I use the flavored body lotions you can buy through adult catalogs. We like the types that feel hot when you lick or blow them. She loves it when I tie her down, blindfold her, and then spread the lotion on her breasts and all over her vagina. It drives her crazy when I suck her breasts and rub the lotion on her clitoris and G-spot. Sometimes I even alternate between the lotion and an ice cube to really make her scream."* —W. R.

Smaller models are often quieter and less disruptive. I highly recommend a slim, half-inch-diameter G-spot vibrator, about 4–6 inches long such as the "First-time Jelly G-spot" model, available from Lover's Lane (www.loverslane.com) and other adult novelty stores.

A hybrid of the vibrating egg and the G-spot vibrator can be found in a few new models that have a "bullet" mounted on the end of a 6-to-10-inch flexible wand. This can be very beneficial for a woman who wants to stimulate her own G-spot, since the wand's angle can be adjusted to reach her G-spot and the wand's length helps extend her reach.

Other Toys to Have on Hand

Another toy to consider is the "Butterfly," which is designed for clitoral stimulation. These vibrating devices are usually very small and lightweight, and shaped in the form of a butterfly. Many of them have elastic or adjustable leg and waist bands, so they can be used hands-free. For women wishing to self-stimulate their G-spots, or for G-spot-experienced couples who want to enhance their pleasure, these vibrators can be fun toys.

Many women report enjoying a vibrator called the "Jack Rabbit," which has a "rabbit" mounted on the shaft. When the vibrator is inserted into the vagina, the rabbit's ears tickle the clitoris.

Self-stimulation

While toys can be beneficial to a woman for self-stimulation, they are not necessary for enjoying what the G-spot can offer. For many women, the most challenging part of self-stimulating the G-spot is actually reaching it.

Why? The answer is simple. Though self-stimulation may be more comfortable lying down, reaching the G-spot in this position requires a very flexible wrist, long fingers, and a short vagina—an uncommon set of attributes. While a few women can manage to reach the spot and stimulate it while lying in a reclined or supine position, most will find a squatting or sitting position with knees apart more accommodating.

There is a second benefit to the squatting or sitting position. Upon first-time stimulation of the G-spot, in some cases a woman may feel a sudden need to urinate, even if she has recently emptied her bladder. To assuage the worry of accidental urination, I recommend that women try self-stimulating while squatting in the bathtub or seated over a clean toilet. These positions allow G-spot access without the fear of "accidents." In addition, lubrication can be freely

"My wife uses a vibrator on her clitoris while I massage her G-spot and suck her breasts. Her orgasm is strong enough she sometimes faints afterward. She loves it." —I. P.

applied, again without the worry of creating a mess. (The urge to urinate is addressed further in Chapter 6, Problemshooting.)

When self-stimulating, take as much time as needed to heighten arousal levels. Whether it's reading a sexy story, fantasizing, playing with sex toys, or simply massaging the breasts and body, do whatever is needed to raise your arousal and make you feel that "ache" or "emptiness" within your vagina.

Once the vaginal craving begins to mount, you may begin exploring for the "magic spot" described in the earlier steps. At first touch, the G-spot may produce only mild pleasure. This is normal. However, as you continue to massage the area and it begins to swell, the pleasure should intensify.

Some women report that, while exploring the vagina with a finger, pushing down on the pelvis just above the pelvic bone helps in locating the G-spot. They often report being able to feel the spot between the internal and external fingers. When you believe you've located your special spot, move slowly. Whether you're using one finger or two, I recommend moving your fingers in a slow, lazy circle, as if you were tracing the rim of a nickel. Experiment. Try a light pressure at first, then a firmer touch. Tease yourself as you go. Make it deliciously slow and torturous. And above all, don't overlook the pleasure you feel along the way. Make the journey erotic and pleasing.

6

Problemshooting

Pain or Discomfort

If at any point your lover expresses pain while stimulating her vagina or G-spot, stop the stimulation and schedule an appointment with her gynecologist. Although the G-spot can cause very slight discomfort if massaged when not aroused, it should not cause true pain.

If she expresses feeling minor discomfort, try applying an approved sexual lubricant to prevent irritating the G-spot's surface. Be sure you're not rubbing the surface too vigorously. Also, be sure your fingernails are smooth and cut short.

If she still feels pain or discomfort, she may suffer from a medical condition such as endometriosis, pelvic inflammatory disease, or a host of other potential causes. So a checkup with the gynecologist is in order.

Inability to Reach Orgasm

In rare cases, women simply can't attain the G-spot orgasm. They'll reach a point were they are close, where the waves are building and fading and building and fading, but they simply can't crest over. This may be a physical problem, but it is most likely psychological. If this happens with your lover, the first step is to reassure her that you're there. It's important to remember that she should feel relaxed, comfortable, and emotionally bonded.

Second, if you haven't done so already, pause long enough to lubricate your hand and her vagina. Having ample lubrication can make an enormous difference in the way nerve endings are stimulated, without irritation to skin surfaces.

Third, if you're absolutely sure she can't achieve the G-spot orgasm, but she wants to keep trying, break the "hands-above-the-breast" rule and try massaging or licking/nibbling at the clitoris while you stroke her G-spot. Be patient and understanding. If your attempt at a G-spot orgasm fails, you may wish to help her achieve a traditional clitoral or vaginal orgasm. Retry the G-spot orgasm on another occasion. Afterward, read the section below titled "The Emotional Aspect" and then reread the ten steps to make sure you're following the instructions to the letter. You may even want to discuss G-spot orgasms with your lover. Some women simply won't allow themselves to "lose control" without understanding what's happening to their bodies.

Above all else, remember that orgasms are emotionally driven for most women. Talking, kissing, holding, reassuring, and building trust are each as important as, sometimes more than, the physical stimulus.

The Urge to Urinate

Upon initial stimulation of the G-spot, some women feel a strong and urgent need to urinate. This can be a legitimate need or a "ghost sensation," depending on whether her bladder is full, partially full, or empty.

In the case of a full or partially full bladder, the pressure being applied near the urethra and bladder neck can bring about a genuine need to urinate. However, if the bladder was emptied recently, the sensation may originate from the stimulation and pressure being applied near the urethra and bladder.

> *"At first, my wife had a lot of trouble with the false sensation of needing to urinate when she neared orgasm. We got beyond this by doing it in the shower."*
> —C. H.

Many women report feeling the ghost sensation of a full bladder in the first few incidences of G-spot stimulation. If ignored, the sensation usually abates, and is quickly replaced with erotic sensations. As a general rule, with repeated exposure (and remembering to empty the bladder before intercourse), most women learn to get beyond this unpleasant sensation.

If your lover can't escape feeling the ghost sensation after several attempts at G-spot stimulation, a visit to her physician or gynecologist may be in order.

Orgasm Anxiety

Some couples set themselves up for failure through a condition called orgasm anxiety (OA). This condition occurs when a person tries to force or rush an orgasm and inadvertently inhibits the orgasm from occurring naturally. OA frequently occurs in people displaying certain behavior patterns: goal seekers and performance givers are the two most common.

Our definition of a goal seeker is a person who focuses strictly on achieving orgasm, placing little emphasis on the pleasure to be experienced along the way. Goal seekers often express feelings of sexual frustration if they don't climax during *every* sexual encounter. Feelings of guilt, inadequacy, or selfishness may arise if they need additional stimulation after their partner has already climaxed—and any of these feelings can inhibit orgasm, thus perpetuating the problem.

> *"If you don't succeed the first try, don't give up. It's worth it when it finally happens. And it will eventually happen when she's ready."* —F. S.

Goal seekers who race their partner to orgasm, and rush or try to force the orgasm, may suffer from OA.

Performance givers, on the other hand, are known for faking orgasms. PGs may not feel the need to climax for their own satisfaction, but they feel the need to orgasm to please their partner, or to avoid damaging their partner's ego. Perhaps their partner feels inadequate if the performance giver doesn't climax; if so, a performance giver can develop OA even though they don't require orgasm for their own benefit.

OA is a good subject to discuss candidly with your partner. Don't let goal seeking or performance giving steal your sexual enjoyment. Talk to your partner about ensuring that each of you enjoys more pleasure along the path of lovemaking. Since it's very unlikely that you'll both achieve orgasm at the same moment every time you make love, discuss your feelings about needing or giving stimulation after the other has climaxed. Discuss the importance each of you each places on climax. You may be surprised by what you learn.

He Said/She Said

One common problem between couples is a misinterpretation of the meaning of *foreplay*. This misinterpretation comes about because men often think in physical terms while women often think in emotional terms. For many men, foreplay is the physical actions which preface intercourse: kissing, touching, massage, fondling the breasts, vaginal or clitoral stimulation, cunnilingus. These physical actions "ready" a woman for the "main event": intercourse and orgasm. These men often also look for physical signs such as erection of the nipples or wetness of the vagina as indicators that their partner is ready for intercourse. While these physical signs can be encouraging, it's important that their partner also be emotionally prepared.

For many women, foreplay is primarily *emotional*—the physical stimuli are secondary. Women often view foreplay in wide and encompassing terms. Foreplay may include spending an evening together, talking, watching TV, sharing hopes and desires, slow dancing, or simply holding hands while walking through the mall. The foreplay slowly and naturally escalates into lovemaking.

Consider this example:

Wife: "I'm almost afraid to kiss him. It's like one kiss leads us right to the bedroom."

Husband: *"She always complains that I jump right into it. But I don't. I kiss her, play with her breasts, massage her womanhood, and give her plenty of foreplay before we ever start."*

This example clearly demonstrates the two different perceptions. The wife feels there is no foreplay or intimacy because there was no emotional bonding prior to their physical contact. To her, the husband jumps right into sex, because he is starting at the point she perceives as only the threshold of lovemaking.

On the other hand, the husband is frustrated because he perceives his wife's need for foreplay as a need for physical stimulus, and he feels he has tried to fulfill that need through kissing her, massaging her breasts, and other forms of petting.

If any of this strikes home with you, be happy about it. Recognizing and accepting the problem is 95 percent of resolving it. What's important to realize is we can't glorify one of these needs—the emotional and the physical—while condemning the other. Neither can be deemed right or wrong. They are simply different.

If you sense there may be confusion about foreplay in your relationship, have a candid chat with your partner about her needs. Be sure to share your needs with her, too. You may be surprised to learn how easily you can accommodate each other's needs while incidentally enriching and deepening your relationship. Even if you don't feel there's a problem in your relationship, it may help to "shoot down" any troubles before they arise.

The Emotional Aspect

Among the women we've polled, the leading impediment to achieving orgasm (of any type) is identified as a "*lack of emotional intimacy*" within the relationship. In a later study we conducted, when women were asked "What is it about sex that gives you the most pleasure?" the leading answer was "emotional intimacy; sharing feelings with a loved one." (This is especially true of performance givers, since their motive for intercourse is emotional bonding rather than pleasure or orgasm.)

While other answers such as "touching and sensuality" and "to achieve orgasm" ranked a close second and third, subjects such as "pleasing him," "cunnilingus," "clitoral massage," "fellatio," and "the excitement" ranked farther down the scale.

These studies reveal two very simple truths: (1) the lack of a needed emotional intimacy can prevent many women from climaxing; and (2) emotional intimacy is the engine driving most women's desire for intercourse.

If your lover is unable to achieve a G-spot orgasm, the most likely cause is her inability to reach a deep level of comfort with the relationship. This is one of those difficult truths that most of us don't want to face, since it pains our ego. But it's better to bear the pain and face the truth than to lie to ourselves, only to have the ugly truth rear it's head again later.

Whether your relationship is new or old, there is always hope. The efforts you have put forth will not go unrewarded. If your relationship is new, it may be that she hasn't yet established a comfortable level of bonding with you. Perhaps she has reservations left over from a previous relationship where she was hurt or felt used. Be patient. Earn her trust.

The positive fact is, even if your partner wasn't able to achieve a G-spot orgasm, you've lavished a wonderful evening on her that will certainly leave a favorable and romantic impression. She'll undoubtedly greet you with a wide smile the next time you meet.

> *"The key to success is the presence of romance. It's much easier to orgasm when you're feeling loved and connected with your partner."* —A. P.

If your relationship is more established, you may have overwhelmed your partner with an uncharacteristic amount of tenderness and bonding. She may have been expecting you to "drop a bomb" at any moment and simply couldn't completely relax. This is especially true if sex has recently been a ritual.

So what are you waiting for? Talk to your partner. If you enjoyed the evening, tell her so. Ask how she enjoyed it. If you both agree that you enjoyed the evening, this is the perfect opportunity to plan your next date. Chances are, next time she'll be more relaxed and you'll succeed.

7

The Same Thing, Only Different

While the ten-step technique has proven effective for most people, it's important to recall that we are individuals, and each of us has different likes and dislikes. We have distinct perceptions of life, personal experiences, our own spiritual views, and subtle idiosyncrasies that make us unique. Like snowflakes falling from a winter sky, we are the same when viewed collectively, yet individual when examined more closely. We are who we are, and no one is exactly the same as anyone else.

Because of this, I encourage you to adapt the ten-step technique to best serve your needs and those of your partner. Carve your own niche. Be creative and adventurous. Make it upbeat and fun. Be romantic and spontaneous. But above all, be the person your partner fell in love with. Be the unique person you are. Adapt what you can and enhance your G-spot experience, just like this couple did:

> *"My wife and I both work corporate jobs. After working ten hours a day, fighting traffic during frantic commutes to and from work then getting through supper, housework yard work, and putting up with the*

day-to-day headaches of life, my wife and I are exhausted by late evening. By 8:00 p.m., we're both ready to sit back, relax, unwind, then go to bed so we can do the whole thing over again the next day. Often, we're too tired to even make love.

Because of this, on our 'date night' l surprised my wife with a special treat. On Friday morning, I sent her flowers at work with a note to expect a 'very special and romantic' evening at home. I took the afternoon off, cleaned the house, made some preparations, and had a candlelight dinner waiting when she walked in from work. After the dinner, I prepared a hot bath and loaded the bathroom with scented candles. While she soaked and relaxed in the tub, I cleaned the kitchen, put on soft music in the bedroom, lit more candles there, and sprinkled the bed with rose petals. When she finished her bath, I led her to the bedroom and gave her a full-body massage with her favorite aromatherapy oils. I started with her back, then the backs of her legs, then her feet. I spent an hour or more just massaging and teasing her It was a great turn-on for both of us. By the time I finished the massage, she was relaxed and in a casual state. The atmosphere was romantic, and we were both aroused and in a sexually comfortable state. It was the perfect lead-in to the latter steps of your technique. From there, everything happened naturally." —J.P.

8

An Interview with
Dr. Beverly Whipple

According to Merriam-Webster's, the word *philanthropy* is defined as "active effort to promote human welfare; a charitable act or gift, (or) goodwill to fellowmen." A related notion, and a common synonym for philanthropy, is *altruism*, defined simply as "an unselfish act performed for the welfare of others." The subject of this interview, Dr. Beverly Whipple, displays both of these admirable characteristics. Dr. Whipple—Ph.D., R.N., FAAN, and a Professor Emeritus of Rutgers University—is one of the world's foremost authorities on the G spot, if not the leading authority, and she was among the group who initially named it.

While I worked with a number of very helpful and friendly doctors, researchers, and sexologists during the writing and compiling of this book, none was more helpful than Dr. Whipple. She unselfishly donated her time and effort to insure that readers of this book received accurate information.

AUTHOR: I'd like to begin the interview by thanking you on behalf of myself and readers for sharing your time and your wealth of knowledge. Your unselfish generosity is com-mendable.

DR. WHIPPLE: You're welcome.

AUTHOR: The first question I wish to pose is a preface to the overall G spot experience: What elements do you feel are important for a woman to achieve a G spot orgasm?

DR. WHIPPLE: A woman has to be comfortable with her body, comfortable and willing to communicate with her partner, and has to be willing to experiment with different positions of sexual intercourse. Acceptance of self is very important. A woman also has to be aware that she is responsible for her own orgasm, and no one can give her an orgasm.

AUTHOR: If we can, let's break that down a little more by examining an "orgasm." Exactly what is an orgasm?

DR. WHIPPLE: It's important to distinguish that in men, or-gasm and ejaculation are two different phenomena and are controlled by two separate nerve pathways. We are just be-ginning to learn more about the neurophysiology of sexual response and sexual behavior in women. As individuals, we say we know what an orgasm is, but I'm not sure we know what it is. In layman's terms, there's a stimulation of nerve pathways, a buildup of tension, and then a release of mus-cle tension. And you do not have to have physical stimula-tion for orgasm to occur. This can also occur with mental stimulation.

AUTHOR: With that in mind, how do G spot orgasms differ from clitoral or vaginal orgasms?

DR. WHIPPLE: There are physiological differences in that with stimulation of the G spot, the uterus pushes down into the vagina, the introitis of the vagina opens and there is a bearing down sensation. With stimulation of the clitoris, the uterus pulls up, the end of the vagina balloons out, and there are contractions in the outer third of the vagina. Women report that an orgasm from G spot stimulation feels deeper inside, whereas an orgasm from clitoral stimulation is more localized in the genital area.

AUTHOR: Do you feel that female ejaculations and the G spot coincide?

DR. WHIPPLE: Not necessarily. In some women they are correlated, in others they are not. In one of the early research articles published on this, research showed a test subject had ejaculation from clitoral stimulation and from G spot stimulation.

AUTHOR: Do all women ejaculate?

DR. WHIPPLE: Most women do have some expulsion of fluid from the ducts and glands into the urethra. And this can occur during clitoral stimulation or vaginal stimulation or G spot stimulation. The fluid goes either into the bladder or out of the urethra as ejaculation. This has been documented by Dr. Francesco Cabello of Malaga, Spain.

AUTHOR: What is known of the fluid women expel during an ejaculation—where is it stored, what is its chemical makeup?

DR. WHIPPLE: It comes from the female prostate gland, which surrounds the urethra and has ducts into the urethra. It is made up of glucose, fructose, PSA, and PAP.

AUTHOR: What health benefits or risks surround G spot orgasms?

DR. WHIPPLE: The obvious benefit is it feels good. Risks could be that someone trying to find it could cause trauma to tissue with long fingernails or improper stimulation or not getting feedback from the woman. Also, stimulation of this area produces a strong natural pain-blocking effect.

AUTHOR: About how far inside the vagina is the G spot?

DR. WHIPPLE: The G spot is found about halfway between the back of the pubic bone (which is on the roof of the vagina) and the cervix, and it's along the course of the urethra. You have to push into the upper vaginal wall to feel this area as it swells. Use a "come here" motion with your fingers to stimulate the area.

It's really hard for women to feel it on themselves unless they have a short vagina and long fingers, because you have to bend down, push up, and push in—although there are instructions on how to find it on yourself. It is difficult to say how far inside the vagina you have to feel because the G spot is felt through the upper vaginal wall, not on it, and each woman is different.

An Interview with Dr. Beverly Whipple

AUTHOR: What would you tell people about finding the G spot?

DR. WHIPPLE: I don't want to see people set up on finding the G spot, or male multiple orgasms, or female ejaculation, or imagery orgasm as a goal they have to achieve. We're all unique individuals. We all have different tastes in terms of the clothing we choose to wear, the foods we choose to eat, the people we choose to be with. I think it's only natural that we have different tastes in what we like sexually. And some women may not find this area sensitive or erotic. Or it may be that someone is not pressing hard enough on the area, because you have to use quite a bit of pressure pushing up through the vaginal wall to feel the area swell. Or they may have long fingernails or rough skin that causes the women to feel uncomfortable.

What's important is we need to be open and aware and help people find whatever is pleasurable for them, whether that be G spot stimulation, clitoral stimulation, or stimulation of other erotic areas. And more importantly, we should enjoy the overall experience and what's felt along the way, not just focusing on achieving an orgasm.

What we need to do is enjoy the experience, not just strive for an orgasm.

AUTHOR: What would help women to learn more about themselves?

DR. WHIPPLE: Men are given permission to touch their penis when they urinate. But for women it's more difficult. Many women get the message as a young child: "Don't touch down there." And it's very difficult for these women to learn about their own bodies because they have been given negative messages about touching their genitals. And you can't learn about yourself without exploring and touching other parts of your body. So women need to learn to be comfortable touching their body for pleasure.

AUTHOR: What will happen if all women become orgasmic?

DR. WHIPPLE: There's so much more to sensuality and sexuality than orgasm. And women are often orgasmic now. But that's not the end-all. That is not it. It's the relationship, the communication, the caring, and the intimacy that are so important. And don't be threatened by a woman's sexuality and sensuality, she's going to enjoy it and you enjoy her enjoying it.

AUTHOR: What can people do to increase their sexual response?

DR. WHIPPLE: I think it's important for women to be aware that they can take control and do some things that will help themselves, not only in terms of mapping their bodies and being aware of what provides them with pleasure. They can use the Kegel exercises. The Kegel exercises are those that are sometimes taught around the time of childbirth, before or after, to increase the strength of the PC muscle. By increasing the strength of this muscle, we find that there is a positive correlation with how strong that muscle is and a woman's orgasmic response. That is, women who have very weak muscles usually don't have orgasms, where women who have particularly strong muscles often have multiple orgasms. This was documented by Graber and Klein Graber in the 1970s.

To identify the muscle to use with the Kegel exercises, become aware of the muscle you use to cut off the flow of urine. You may want to test the strength of your pubococcygeus or PC muscle before you start the exercise program. Put two fingers into the vagina, yours or your partners, open them up like scissors, and then try to close them with your muscles. Don't be surprised if you cannot do that.

Start off the exercises slowly, contracting and relaxing the muscles you use to cut off the flow of urination, slowly building up the repetitions to 100 times per day. Then, in a month, repeat the test by inserting two fingers into the vagina and trying to squeeze the fingers together to see if the muscle is getting stronger. This is a good way for women to take control of their health and their sexual response.

Not only is it good for women to do, they are also good for men. Men can do the same exercise to increase sexual pleasure and orgasm. Men have reported that their erections are stronger after strengthening the PC muscle. By increasing the strength of this muscle and then squeezing the muscle at the moment of ejaculatory inevitability, some men can learn to have multiple orgasms through preventing ejaculation. Here again, it's important to realize that ejaculation and orgasm are two separate phenomena and need not occur simultaneously.

AUTHOR: If a woman does Kegel exercises, will her vagina be tighter?

DR. WHIPPLE: It may become tighter. As the strength of the PC muscle increases she may feel tighter during vaginal intercourse. And also, a very good way of doing the exercise is with a penis inside the vagina. You're then doing the exercises against a resistance device, which is always more effective. And also, the male will have pleasure and enjoyment from the stimulation of the penis by the PC muscle.

AUTHOR: How can a man test the strength of his PC muscle?

DR. WHIPPLE: There's a very fun way for men to test the strength of their PC muscles. First of all, you want to do this in private. When you start out, before you do the exercise, put a tissue over an erect penis and lift it up. And most men will smile and say "I can do that," but that's a pretty weak muscle. So after they do the exercise for a month or so—the same as the women do by contracting then relaxing the muscle that stops the flow of urination—they can try the test again. Then, they may try doing the test with a washcloth, and then a hand towel, and eventually a wet hand towel. This is just to test the strength of the muscle. The exercise is for fun and sexual enjoyment.

AUTHOR: What affect does aging have on sexual response?

DR. WHIPPLE: There are some physiological changes during the aging process. Men and women may take a little longer as they get older to become sexually aroused. It may take longer for men to have an erection and may take longer for ejaculation. For women, it may take longer to have vaginal lubrication. Also, women may not have as many contractions as they once did, and the contractions may not be as strong. But instead of comparing the process to how it was, it is important to enjoy sensual and sexual as it is. Here again, the Kegel exercises can help in keeping sexuality more vital.

AUTHOR: In closing, I'd like to thank you once again for sharing your knowledge with readers. It is appreciated and I'm sure readers can benefit from the information you've provided.

9

Case Studies

Female Responses

Subject A *Age: 49; marital status:* married/divorced/
         remarried

Subject B *Age: 32; marital status:* married

Subject C *Age: 25; marital status:* single, engaged

Prior to you (or your mate) having read this book, had you experienced a G-spot orgasm?

Female Subject A: No.

Female Subject B: No.

Female Subject C: I'd never felt anything like it.

Before your first G-spot experience, did you climax on a regular basis through intercourse?

Female Subject A: Yes and no. During my first marriage, I never climaxed and hated having sex. My ex-husband was rough, selfish, and impatient. Sex with him was painful and never a source of pleasure for me. It was the sore point of our marriage. He called me "frigid" and he didn't understand why I never enjoyed sex. He acted as if something was wrong with me, and after hearing it over and over, I began to believe him. I tried talking to my mother and grandmother about the problem, but found no support. They presented sex as the duty of a "good wife" in fulfilling her husband's needs and as a means of procreating.

The first time I made love with my present husband, it was a totally new experience. He's patient and gentle, and I climaxed several times the first night we made love. It was a true awakening and gave me a sense of renewed self-confidence. It made me realize that I wasn't "frigid"—there wasn't anything wrong with me—and I wasn't solely responsible for the first failed marriage. Now, I nearly always climax. When I feel my husband beginning to swell inside me, it throws me right over the edge. And on the rare occasions when he climaxes before I do, he helps me achieve orgasm by either continuing to move, oral stimulation, or with sexual props. We never have a problem because we talk openly and I don't end up feeling "rushed."

Female Subject B: No. I can sometimes climax when my husband orally stimulates my clitoris or uses a vibrator, but can't [climax] with just his penis. I need lots of cuddling and loving beforehand to get me in a sensual mood.

Female Subject C: Not every time. It depended on the guy— how I felt about him and my mood when it happened.

How much did you enjoy sex before your first G-spot orgasm?

Female Subject A: With my second husband, I've always enjoyed making love.

Female Subject B: That's a hard question to answer. Our sex life was good, but nothing like it is now. I guess I felt that something was missing—like there should be deeper pleasure and intensity—do you understand what I mean?

("Yes. . .")

"I'd find myself reading romance novels and dreaming of someday feeling the kind of pleasure those women feel. But I wasn't sure if that was real or merely the yearnings of fiction.

Female Subject C: Sometimes I enjoyed it; other times, if I really liked a certain guy, it was an easy way to deepen the relationship.

Can you describe the first time you experienced a G-spot orgasm?

Female Subject A: Yes. I'll never forget it. But where should I begin? Okay. Let's see. I'd have to say my husband blindsided me with it. He never gave me a single clue that he'd read the book or what he was planning. He just asked me out on a "date"—and considering that we're married, I felt that his "asking me out" was flattering. It was a very romantic gesture and I was looking forward to making it up to him, come date night.

When our "date" finally rolled around, he surprised me by coming home from work with a dozen roses. We went out to dinner (which I loved because I didn't have to cook or do cleanup afterward). Then after dinner, we went for a moonlight stroll, then came home and cuddled on the sofa while watching a movie.

I guess I was aroused because I had been looking forward to "making it up to him" all week. And he was aroused too, probably by his secret agenda. We ended up necking through most of the movie—just like we were teenagers—until we got home and I was so ready I stripped off my clothes and most of his. I wanted him then and there.

Instead, he picked me up and carried me to the bedroom, laid me on the bed, finished undressing, and began kissing me all over again.

In retrospect, having read the book now, I can see how he was following the steps. But he was also concentrating his attention on me, and I could feel it. His attention was focused much deeper than our regular lovemaking. We had a connection going. It was almost spiritual. And even though I was ready for him at any moment, I didn't feel rushed, and loved what he was doing to me.

He nuzzled and sucked my breasts until I felt like my whole body was yearning for him. And by the time he finally touched me, I thought I would explode. It was like tuning guitar strings, tweaking them tighter and tighter until you just know that the next turn of the knob they're going to go. I can remember pushing and thrusting against his hand, begging him to massage me, yet loving the way he was teasing me.

When he finally entered me with his finger and began massaging my G-spot, the tension drained from me and I felt like I was floating in the clouds. It was relaxing to have that hungry void filled, while I was still highly aroused. I'm not really sure how to describe it. It's like hot and cold. He was sucking and teasing my breasts, which made me yearn.

But his finger was fulfilling the void with every new yearning. It was heaven.

A few minutes into it, I could tell something totally new was happening inside me. I don't know how to describe it, but I could feel an orgasm building and knew it would be much deeper and much more intense than anything I'd ever felt before. There was a great sense of building. I can't put it into words. It was scary. I wanted it to happen yet I knew I'd have to let myself go completely to reach it. And that was hard to do. I didn't want to make a fool of myself in front of my husband, thrashing around or screaming. At the same time, I was afraid he'd stop what he was doing and I'd be terribly disappointed.

He must have felt me tense up or something at that very moment—maybe it was the connection we had. . . I don't know—but he said exactly what I needed to hear. He told me: "Don't worry. I'm here. I know what's happening to you. I love you. Just relax and let it happen."

And I did. I could feel it building inside of me, like waves, each a little higher than the last. He continued telling me how much he loved me and reassuring me. I'm not sure how he was able to talk because I never felt his mouth leave my breasts, but he did it somehow.

A couple of times I peaked out really high and was close to cresting over. I wanted it to happen so badly, yet was afraid it wouldn't, and part of me was a little wary of it. But after the third or fourth peak—just when I started to think I wasn't going to make it—I felt this warmth start inside of me, spreading outward from my core. I could feel it building and building and building and I realized then, even if I wanted to stop it, I couldn't.

When it finally came I screamed and was squinting my eyes closed so hard that I could see red. I could feel myself contracting hard against his finger, trying to suck it in, getting warmer and tighter and warmer and tighter. It was by far the best thing I'd ever felt—better than I imagined. I don't really have words to describe it. It just felt so good and kept going and going much longer than any orgasm I'd ever had. It was so warm and so deep. I wanted it to last forever.

After what seemed like an eternity (which my husband later told me was two and a half minutes), it began to fade. I became vaguely aware that the bed and the inside of my thighs were very wet. For a minute, I wondered if I had lost control and peed the bed during the climax—but I forgot about that as my husband quickly removed his finger and inserted himself inside of me. He was obviously highly aroused, was rock hard, and began swelling almost instantly. His penis felt about three times its normal size and he was marveling about how tight I was. He came right away and his swelling threw me right over the edge again and we climaxed together.

After we laid together panting for a few minutes and floated back down to earth, I realized that the bed actually was wet. Very wet. It was absolutely drenched. I felt certain I had lost control of myself and was very embarrassed. That first time was the wettest I've ever been. But he assured me I hadn't peed, that a stream of clear fluid had shot out of me and was gushing past his hand and splattering between my knees.

I would say I was skeptical, but skeptical may not be a precise description of what I felt. I think "wonderment" is a more appropriate term. I was astonished, stunned, and curious at the same time. I had to examine some of the fluid on my thighs just to reassure myself. It didn't smell like urine and was clear, with just a hint of milkiness. And it was slick—not as slick as my normal lubricant, but not nearly as sticky as urine.

Afterward, he explained how he had come across the book and how it had piqued his curiosity. He showed me the book and we read parts of it and talked about how women have the ability to ejaculate (as I had).

I've got to admit, I loved him more right then than I ever remember loving anything. What he did for me—for us—was so selfless. And since then, our relationship has never been stronger.

Female Subject B: Not in a single word. It was the best thing I've ever felt.

("Better than other orgasms you'd had?")

Oh, yes, by a long shot. In the past, when my husband made love to me, I'd get really keyed up about the time he was ready to go to sleep. The problem was, as soon as he came, the "show was over. I don't want you to get the wrong idea here—I love my husband dearly and enjoy making love with him—but it was frustrating to watch him have such a fulfilling orgasm and then fade off to sleep while I was left tossing and turning and wanting more.

On some nights I'd feel satisfied. Other times, one or two orgasms just weren't enough for me. The problem wasn't the quantity of orgasms, it was the quality. The depth. The orgasms I had with my husband (and other men before my marriage) just weren't deep enough. They left me sensing there should be more, which ties in with what I mentioned earlier about the romance novels and wanting to feel the deep satisfaction those fictional women feel.

After that first G-spot orgasm, I knew I'd found what I was missing. I felt completely satisfied afterward. I was drained [laughs]—literally.

Female Subject C: Intense pleasure. That's the only way I know how to describe it. It was very different from anything I'd felt. As strange as it sounds, I'm glad it hadn't happened earlier in my life because I wouldn't have anything to compare it to.

After your first G-spot experience, has it been easier or harder for you to achieve G-spot orgasms? And how do they compare to the first experience?

Female Subject A: The second time my husband tried the technique it took longer for me to climax. I had a really hard time reaching it and ended up "giving up" before it finally happened. I think my husband had relaxed a little and wasn't following all of the steps to the letter—and in some ways, that was a reversion back to our previous lovemaking.

Not that it was bad before. I just wanted to feel his focus and the emotional bond we had the first time.

Part of the problem was my own, too. I wanted to feel the climax so badly that I tried to rush it. But I've since learned that this isn't something you can make happen. Every time I tried to force it to happen, it faded away just when I was ready to crest over. It reminded me of a wanderer in the desert chasing a mirage. You know? The faster you run after it, the farther away it gets.

After getting really, really close five or six times, I gave up. I began to cry because I was afraid that the first time had been a fluke and I'd never get to feel another climax like that first one again. Plus, my husband had been caressing the spot for about 45 minutes and I was feeling guilty and selfish. I knew he wanted to climax, too, and I figured his hand was getting tired and was probably hurting. It was frustrating and made me see the wisdom behind your advising people [in the book] not to tell the woman about it beforehand. Once you know how good it's going to be, the apprehension is almost painful and can be inhibiting."

("Did you eventually reach the climax?")

Yes. I told my husband that I couldn't make it and asked him to stop. By then, I'd given up completely. I was very disappointed. He stopped caressing my G-spot and started caressing my breasts and abdomen while we talked. He told me that I was probably trying too hard and I just needed to try to relax and let it happen naturally. I remember telling him that I couldn't relax because I wanted it to happen too badly, but was afraid it would never happen again. I also told him I was feeling guilty for how long it was taking, and he told me not to feel guilty, that he enjoyed seeing me feel good. He told me that he loved me and asked me if massaging the G-spot felt good even when I didn't completely make it. I told him yes, and said I loved him, too. He asked if I would let him try again and would just relax and enjoy what I was feeling at the moment instead of focusing on the climax. By then, I was beginning to feel a vaginal yearning again and didn't need much convincing. He teased me a little more and then began caressing my G-spot again. As soon as he touched it, I could feel another wave start building, but instead of trying to make it come, I tried to focus on what I was feeling. Within 30 seconds, I climaxed.

Since then, I've learned not to try to force it to happen. And the more we do it, the easier it is for me. We've done it standing in the shower, on the washing machine during the spin cycle, the couch; anyplace works fine.

Female Subject B: I had a few slow times at first. I had to be lying down and had to make myself relax. But after the first few times it got faster and easier. And now I can ejaculate right away and can do it in other positions. Once we did it while standing in the shower. And sometimes now I have a G-spot orgasm when I take the top during regular lovemaking. It's never been as good as the first time it happened, but it's come close and it's still more fulfilling than other orgasms. You won't hear me complaining.

Female Subject C: It keeps getting better and better.

Male Responses

Subject A *Age: 38; marital status:* married
Subject B *Age: 34; marital status:* married
Subject C *Age: 27; marital status:* single, engaged

Did you succeed on your first attempt to give a G-spot orgasm?

Male Subject A: Yes.

Male Subject B: No.

Male Subject C: Yes.

Approximately how long did it take from the beginning of the actual G-spot stimulation until the orgasm began?

Male Subject A: The first time took about 45 minutes. About 30 minutes into it, my forearm started burning and lightly cramping. It wasn't overly painful, but it was enough to cause doubts about the system and my wife's "supposed" ability to have a G-spot orgasm. However, I could tell something was happening with my wife by the way she was moaning and moving and telling me not to stop. I figured, if nothing else, it was a great workout for the muscles in my forearm and a thorough test for the system if I could keep it up a few more minutes. By the 40-minute mark, my arm felt like it was on fire and I was having trouble keeping my finger movement steady. This worked out for the best because, by then, my wife had started urging me to go faster. I could

see the desperation in her eyes and I wanted to go faster—
and would have if I could—but my forearm muscles would-
n't allow it. It was the agonizingly slow pace that pushed
her right over the edge. Had I moved faster or harder, I would
have delayed her climax without realizing it.

The second time took a while, too. But since then
we've gotten faster and faster at bringing the climax about.
Now, we can often do it within 5 minutes. We can use
other positions and I can often insert myself just before it
happens so we climax together.

Male Subject B: 20 minutes.

Male Subject C: 25–30 minutes.

Have you always succeeded?

Male Subject A: About 99 percent of the time.

Male Subject B: Ah . . . no. I'm embarrassed to mention this,
but when I first got the book I didn't read it. I scanned
through it, looked at the diagram, and tried stimulating my
wife's G-spot the next time we had sex. When I asked her
how it was feeling she said it was "different" and "unusual"
and "it felt good" but nothing seemed to be happening.
She kept guiding my hand back to her clitoris, so I stopped
and figured the whole thing was a hoax.

A few days later I got to work early and my boss called
on the cell phone and said he'd be running about half an
hour late. It was about 20 degrees outside and since I did-
n't have a key to get inside, it meant I'd have to wait in the
car until he got there. I have to wonder if there wasn't some

divine intervention going on because I'd hidden the book under the car seat and had nothing better to do than read it. The funny thing is, I finished the last page just as my boss turned into the parking lot.

As I read the book, I realized the mistakes I'd made and figured it was worth another try, this time following the steps instead of trying to muddle my way through it.

It went like clockwork. Since then, my wife has G-spot orgasms every time I use the technique and our relationship has never been stronger.

Male Subject C: Most of the time. I think it depends on the girl.

What was the most extraordinary or remarkable thing you learned from this book?

Male Subject A: I didn't know my wife had the ability to ejaculate before I read the book. I thought only a few women could "squirt" (as they call it) and guessed these women had some type of physical anomaly which allowed the squirting. It made them perfect candidates for porn movies.

Now I've learned the opposite is true of what I believed. From the book, I've learned that most women have this inherent capacity. And it's amazing that so many people are still unaware of it. Totally unbelievable.

Male Subject B: Before I read the book, I thought the whole G-spot thing was a hoax. I thought that my wife did ejaculate when she achieved orgasm and it was a small amount that mixed right in with her natural lubrication. I'm glad I was wrong! The first time she had a G-spot orgasm she drenched the bed. We were in bed with the lights off, so I couldn't see the fluid coming out of her. But I could feel my hand and the bed getting soaked. And later, when we turned on the lights to change the sheets, there was about a foot-wide wet circle where she was lying. I was shocked that all the G-spot stuff was true.

Male Subject C: The whole thing, the strength of the orgasm and the ejaculation. The first time I did it, I was with a girl-friend I'd been dating off and on for about four months. We'd had sex a few times and it was good, but not great. She was always quiet during sex and would just lie there motionless and moan a little bit. And then afterward, she would act like I owed her some big favor. But that first night [using the G-spot technique] was wild and different! At first she just started moaning like usual. But her moans kept getting louder and louder and she started saying "Oh, God, don't stop! Oh, God, don't stop!" over and over. Then she started bucking and gasping and kept getting louder and louder until she was screaming it. I was loving it! I half expected the cops to show up at any minute because the walls in my apartment are paper-thin. But she didn't seem to care, she kept screaming. She looked like she was in la-bor and was giving birth. Then she went dead silent and was really straining and all this fluid started kind of bub-bling and flowing out of her. It was awesome. She followed me around like a puppy for a week afterward and wanted to do it all day and night.

What do you enjoy most about G-spot orgasms?

Male Subject A: Wow. That's a tough question. There's more than one answer. For one thing, I like seeing the pleasure my wife is experiencing and knowing that I provided that pleasure for her. It's very satisfying and it lends a certain sense of both love and power. But it runs deeper than just that. Before I learned this technique, when my wife would climax I never had distinct physical signs to go by. She could have easily faked it and I'd have no way of knowing differently. I simply had to take her word for it. There were no distinct guideposts. When she neared a climax, her breathing would increase. I might feel a very slight tightening in her vagina and her moaning would grow louder, but that was it. There was never a clear beginning or end.

Now all the doubt is gone. I have undeniable physical signs to go by. As she starts the climax, her vagina begins constricting and squeezing against my finger so tightly that it threatens to force my finger out! She's so tight and wet and warm that it drives me crazy. And then the fluid comes and her moans turn to screams. There's simply no more doubt about when the climax begins and when it ends.

Male Subject B: This technique has truly revitalized my marriage. My wife and I are closer and more open now than we've ever been before. Our sex life is great and our relationship is stronger than ever.

Our relationship changed drastically the first time she had the G-spot orgasm. I think it comes down to trust. When it was happening, I realized that it was so extremely intense for her that she was putting all of her trust in me, completely. She had to let go fully and shed all inhibitions in order to reach it. By doing that, she was handing me the reins of control. She was giving me all the power and trusting that I wouldn't abuse it or make fun of her afterward or let harm come to her while it was happening. And that even though she wasn't sure what was physically happening to her, she trusted me to guide her through it.

When I realized just how much trust she was showing, it touched me deeply. All the barriers that life had silently erected between us crumbled. There was a new connection between us. As new age as it sounds, there was a oneness. There was complete trust. And now that we've developed this trust, we're free to play and try new things without fear of recrimination. We don't have all the inhibitions and reservations we had before. We've taken our relationship to a higher plane.

Male Subject C: A lot of things. Seeing women squirt and writhe and go crazy with the pleasure. Feeling them get so wet and tight as they convulse against your finger. It really boosts a man's self-confidence. You don't have to wonder if you're better in bed than the last guy she was with, you know? Unless he knows this technique, you know you're better. And you can usually tell right away, afterward.

Did your lover know she could ejaculate?

Male Subject A: No. She was stunned afterward.

Male Subject B: Are you kidding? She couldn't believe it. I had to show her the book to convince her that she hadn't lost control and wet the bed.

Male Subject C: Mostly no.

How much fluid does your lover normally produce when she ejaculates?

Male Subject A: If you want an average, I'd guess she produces somewhere between a tablespoonful and half a cup. Although, the first time, it seemed like at least a cupful, maybe more.

To be honest I haven't found any rhyme or reason to the amount she ejaculates. Sometimes the fluid gushes out of her and other times it's little more than a trickle and hardly noticeable. It doesn't seem to coincide with the intensity of her orgasm, either.

You know, I guess the same is true with men if you think about it. I mean, the amount varies and the projection varies. Sometimes we can shoot for two or three feet while other times the sperm just spurts out of us.

Male Subject B: The first time I did it to her, it was a lot. We didn't measure it, but she drenched the bed so much that we had to change the sheets. Since then, the amount has varied. Some nights she really drenches the bed and some nights it just kind of oozes out of her.

Male Subject C: Women put men to shame. They say that men usually make about a teaspoonful of sperm. But most of the women I've tried this technique on drench the bed. I'd say it's usually a cupful.

What other comments can you share with us?

Male Subject A: I'm still in awe of the G-spot. It amazes me that I've been sexually active for 21 years now—since I was 17—yet I never found the G-spot. Considering that I had several girlfriends before I got married, plus 15 years of marriage and having sex two or three times a week, it just boggles my mind that I—we—never came across it! And now that I know it exists, it's almost embarrassing to think that it's been there all along. It's incredible because I can see how I could have passed through my whole life without ever knowing about it, had you not shared your information in this book.

Male Subject B: Your technique has changed my life and my marriage for the better. Thank you. You don't know what a difference you've made in our lives.

Male Subject C: I wish you would stop selling this book so other guys wouldn't find out about it.

10

The Climax

Pat yourself on the back. Whether or not your first attempt at the G-spot orgasm is successful, you've done two great things. You've spent a little time and money to unselfishly help your partner feel the ultimate in female pleasure—a noble act indeed—and you've made an investment in yourself, gaining knowledge that you can carry throughout life, knowledge you can use time and time again to deliver the ultimate female orgasm.

Questionnaire

A Study of the G-Spot

To aid us and your partner in making strides in G-spot orgasms, we encourage all readers to complete the following survey or mail any personal comments or questions. Mail should be directed to:

Donald L. Hicks

c/o Amorata Press

P.O. Box 3440

Berkeley, CA 94703

Part 1

This part to be completed by the person who applies the G-spot stimulation

Your age: _____

Your sex: M / F

Race:

- ○ White
- ○ Asian
- ○ Native American

- ○ Black
- ○ Hispanic
- ○ Other _____

1. Did you read the entire book?

    yes / no

    • If you answered no, which part did you not read, and why?

_____

_____

_____

_____

2. What was the most extraordinary or remarkable thing you learned from this book?

_____

_____

_____

_____

3. Before reading the book, were you aware of the G-spot's location?

    yes / no

4. Were you aware that women can ejaculate?

    yes / no

5. Did you find the book easy to follow?

    yes / no

6. Can you suggest any way to improve the book?

_____

_____

_____

_____

7. Was your first attempt at applying the G-spot orgasm successful?

   yes / no
   - If not, how many attempts did you make? _____
   - Did you eventually succeed? yes / no

8. If you succeeded (on any attempt), did your lover ejaculate?

   yes / no

9. If your lover ejaculated, how much fluid did she produce?
   - ○ a trickle
   - ○ about a teaspoonful
   - ○ a tablespoonful
   - ○ a cup
   - ○ She drenched the bedsheets

10. Approximately how long did it take from the start of actual G-spot stimulation until the orgasm began?

    _____ hours   _____ minutes

11. Approximately how long did the orgasm last?

    _____ minutes

12. Was your lover surprised by the intensity of the orgasm?

    yes / no

13. Was your lover surprised to learn she could ejaculate?

    yes / no

14. Which of the following choices best match
    your lover's reaction after the orgasm? (choose
    up to three)
    - O joyous/elated
    - O loving/romantic
    - O embarrassed
    - O ready for more
    - O surprised
    - O curious
    - O thankful
    - O frustrated
    - O shy
    - O satiated/fulfilled
    - O angry
    - O other: _____

What other comments can you share with us?

_____

_____

_____

_____

Part 2

*This part to be completed by the woman who
receives the G-spot stimulation*

Your age: _____

Race:

○ White   ○ Black

○ Asian   ○ Hispanic

○ Native American   ○ Other _____

1. Do you typically orgasm during foreplay or intercourse?

   yes / no

2. If you typically orgasm, how many times do you
   normally orgasm (on average) during intercourse
   (foreplay included)?

   ○ 0

   ○ 1–2

   ○ 3–4

   ○ 5–6

   ○ more than 6

3. How long is your typical orgasm?

   ○ Average (8 to 19 seconds)

   ○ Shorter or longer; state duration _____

4. What do you feel is the predominant source of
   orgasm for you?

   ○ Clitoral stimulation

   ○ Vaginal stimulation

   ○ Other: _____

5. Did you experience a "G-spot" orgasm when your partner applied this technique?

    yes / no

6. If yes, how did you feel afterward?
    - ○ joyous/elated
    - ○ loving/romantic
    - ○ embarrassed
    - ○ ready for more
    - ○ surprised
    - ○ curious
    - ○ thankful
    - ○ frustrated
    - ○ shy
    - ○ satiated/fulfilled
    - ○ angry
    - ○ other: _____

7. Did you ejaculate?

    yes / no

8. If yes, did you know prior to the ejaculation that females have the ability to ejaculate?

    yes / no

9. How did this orgasm compare to previous orgasms you've had?

    _____

    _____

    _____

    _____

10. Was there anything you did not like about the G-spot orgasm or the technique your lover used?

_____

_____

_____

_____

11. What other comments can you share?

_____

_____

_____

_____

12. On a scale of 1 to 10, with 1 being least pleasurable and 10 being most pleasurable, how would you rate orgasms you've experienced from the following? (Use 0 if never experienced)
   • Clitoral stimulation: _____
   • Vaginal stimulation: _____
   • G-spot stimulation: _____

All comments gathered through this survey become the property of Hooked on Books. Hooked on Books will not use any names or other information that discloses the identities of the individuals in the survey.

Optional Disclosure

Name: _____

E-mail Address: _____

Address: _____

City: _____ State: _____ Zip: _____

Country: _____

Resources for Further Research

Recommended Reading

The G Spot and Other Discoveries About Human Sexuality, by Alice Kahn Ladas, Beverly Whipple, and John D. Perry. New York: Dell Publishing, 1982; Henry Holt & Company, 2005.

Seduce Me! How to Ignite Your Partner's Passion, by Darcy A. Cole. Universal Publishers, 2003.

The Hite Report: A Nationwide Study of Female Sexuality, by Shere Hite. New York: Dell Publishing Co., Inc., 1976.

The Human Female Prostate, by Milan Zaviacic. Slovak Republic: Slovak Academic Press, 1999.

The G-Spot in Words and Pictures, by Felix G. Berger. Orion-Verlag, 1988.

Secrets of Sensual Lovemaking: The Ultimate in Female Ecstasy, by Tom Leonardi. New York: New American Library (Penguin), 1998.

Websites

SexualHealth.com

This site is a great information resource. It allows visitors to ask questions, browse topics, videos, and products. It also has a board of sexual experts.

The Kinsey Institute
www.indiana.edu/~kinsey

The Kinsey Institute makes available a host of research publications, along with upcoming events and sexology links.

American Association of Sexuality Educators, Counselors, and Therapists (AASECT)
www.aasect.org

A nonprofit professional organization of sexuality educators, sex counselors and sex therapists, AASECT includes among its members physicians, nurses, social workers, psychologists, allied health professionals, clergy members, lawyers, sociologists, marriage and family counselors and therapists, and family planning specialists and researchers, as well as students in relevant professional disciplines. These individuals share an interest in promoting understanding of human sexuality and healthy sexual behavior.

Lover's Lane
www.loverslane.com

Lover's Lane is a tasteful adult resource, geared toward couples. They offer adult books, apparel, and sex toys.

Glossary

analgesic   An agent for producing insensibility to pain.

anterior   Located in the front; the front wall.

blended orgasm   Multiple orgasms occurring simultaneously.

bonding   The act of growing emotionally united.

climax   The highest point; orgasm.

clitoris   A small, highly sensitive organ at the anterior or ventral part of the vulva, homologous to the penis.

elucidate   To make clear by explanation; to bring to light.

female ejaculation   The expulsion of liquid from the urethra by a woman.

female prostate   Also known as the Skene's glands or paraurethral glands; a network of glands and ducts surrounding the urethra and bladder neck.

G-spot   The Gräfenberg Spot. A highly sensitive area located on the anterior wall of the vagina. This spot was named by Dr. Beverly Whipple and Dr. John Perry, after Dr. Ernst Gräfenberg.

G-spot virgin   A woman who has never experienced a G-spot orgasm.

ghost sensation   A false sensation; in the context of this book, a false feeling of the need to urinate.

goal seeker   Individuals who focus on achieving orgasm during each sexual experience and are discontented if orgasm does not occur.

gynecologist   Doctor specializing in diseases and hygiene of women.

hovering   Floating; to be in an uncertain state. In the context of this book, to hold the hand above sensitive areas of the partner's body to create sexual anxiety.

hypothesize   To make an assumption in order to test its validity.

immunohistochemical   Of or relating to the application of histochemical and immunologic methods to chemical analysis of living cells and tissues.

innervate   To supply with nerves; to arouse or stimulate (a nerve or an organ) to activity.

introitus   The orifice of a body cavity; especially, the vaginal opening.

kachapati   A rite of passage reportedly practiced by the Batoro tribe of Africa, through which adolescent girls were taught to "spray the walls" and thus graduate into a state of nubility.

Kegel exercises   Exercises designed to strengthen the pubococcygeus (PC) muscle.

labia   Folds of fatty or vascular flesh bounding the vulva; the lips of the vagina, consisting of the labia majora (outer folds) and labia minora (inner folds).

magic triangle   The area of the genitals covered in pubic hair.

monolithic   Exhibiting solid uniformity, as of a social structure.

obstetricians   Physicians who specialize in pregnancy and childbirth.

orgasm   A climax during sexual excitement.

orgasm anxiety   A condition characterized by chronic fear of not attaining orgasm during intercourse.

paraurethral   Adjacent to the urethra.

performance giver   A person who feels the need to orgasm for the benefit of his or her sexual partner.

physiological   Pertaining to the functional processes of a living organism or any of its parts.

pubococcygeus muscle   A muscle group that acts to help support the pelvic viscera, to draw the lower end of the rectum toward the pubis, and to constrict the rectum and female vagina; also called PC muscle.

retrograde ejaculation   In the context of this work, the ejaculation of fluids backward into the bladder instead of outward from the urethra.

safer sex   Practices minimizing contact with bodily fluids or reducing the risk of contracting sexually transmitted disease.

sexual response   Response to sexual stimulus.

Skene's glands   A small mass of glands and ducts surrounding the urethra; often considered the female prostate glands or paraurethral glands.

stimulation   Arousal, excitement, increasing activity.

urethra   The canal that carries urine out of the bladder; it also serves as a passageway for the ejection of male and female ejaculate.

USI   Urinary stress incontinence. The loss of control or restraint of the bladder.

uterus   The womb; the female organ wherein the fetus develops.

vaginal marksman   A sexual partner whose goal is to initiate vaginal stimulation upon the first permissible opportunity, often in haste.

vulva   The external genital parts of the female.

Endnotes

1. Stoff, J. A., M.D., and Clouatre, D., Ph.D., *The Prostate Miracle: New Natural Therapies That Can Save Your Life* (Kensington Pub. Corp., 2000).

2. Whipple, B., Ph.D., RN, FAAN, and Komisaruk, B. R., Ph.D., "Beyond the G Spot: Recent Research on Female Sexuality," *Psychiatric Annals* 29: 1 (January 1999): 35–57.

3. Singer, I., *The Goals of Human Sexuality* (New York: Norton, 1973); Singer, J., and Singer, I., "Types of Female Orgasm," *Journal of Sex Research* 8 (1972).

4. Ladas, A., Whipple, B., and Perry, J.,*The G Spot and Other Discoveries About Human Sexuality* (Dell Publishing, 1982, reprint, 1983), 140–154.

5. Hite, S., *The Hite Report* (Dell Publishing, 1976), 618.

6. Ogden G., "Perceptions of Touch in Easily Orgasmic Women During Peak Sexual Experiences," (Ph.D. dissertation, Institute for Advanced Study of Human Sexuality, 1981).

7. Whipple, B., Ogden, G., and Komisaruk, B. R., "Physiological Correlates of Imagery Induced Orgasm in

Women," *Archives of Sexual Behavior* 21(2) (1992): 121–133.

8. Ladas, A., Whipple, B., and Perry, J., *The G Spot and Other Discoveries About Human Sexuality* (Dell Publishing, 1982, reprint, 1983), 70–71.

9. Addiego, F., Belzer, E. G., Comolli, J., et al., "Female Ejaculation: A Case Study," *Journal of Sex Research* 17 (1981): 31–21.

10. Zaviacic, M., Dolezalova, S., Holoman, I. K., et al., "Concentrations of Fructose in Female Ejaculate and Urine: A Comparative Biochemical Study," *Journal of Sex Research* 24 (1988): 319–325.

11. Belzer, E. G., Whipple, B., Moger, W., "On Female Ejaculation," *Journal of Sex Research* 20 (1984): 403–406.

12. Sensabaugh, G. R., and Kahane, D., "Biochemical Studies on 'Female Ejaculates,'" presented at the meeting of the California Association of Criminologists, Newport Beach, CA (May 1982).

13. Zaviacic, M., Whipple, B., "Update on the Female Prostate and the Phenomenon of Female Ejaculation," *Journal of Sex Research* 30: 2 (1993): 148–121.

14. Ladas, A., Whipple, B., and Perry, J., *The G Spot and Other Discoveries About Human Sexuality* (Dell Publishing, 1982, reprint, 1983).

15. Addiego, F., Belzer, E. G., Comolli, J., et al., "Female Ejaculation: A Case Study," *Journal of Sex Research* 17 (1981): 31–21.

16. Leonardi, T., *Secrets of Sensual Lovemaking: The Ultimate in Female Ecstasy* (Signet, 1998), 101–103.

17. Ladas, A., Whipple, B., and Perry, J., *The G Spot and Other Discoveries About Human Sexuality* (Dell Publishing, 1982, reprint, 1983), 81.

18. Cabello Santamaria, F., "Female Ejaculation, Myth and Reality," in J. J. Borras-Valls and M. Perez-Conchillo (eds.), *Sexuality and Human Rights* (Proceedings of the XIII World Congress of Sexology, Valencia; NAU, 1998): 325–333.

19. Zaviacic, M., Zaviacicova, A., Holoman, I. K., and Molcan, J., "Female Urethral Expulsions Evoked by Local Digital Stimulation of the G Spot: Differences in the Response Patterns," *Journal of Sex Research* 24 (1988): 311–318.

20. Ladas, A., Whipple, B., and Perry, J., *The G Spot and Other Discoveries About Human Sexuality* (Dell Publishing, 1982, reprint, 1983), 69.

21. Kilbraten, P., personal communication, referenced in Ladas, A., Whipple, B., and Perry, J., *The G Spot and Other Discoveries About Human Sexuality* (Dell Publishing, 1982, reprint, 1983), 75.

22. Muller, J., et al., "The Myocardial Onset Study," *Journal of the American Medical Association* (May 1996).

23. Whipple, B., "Sexual Counseling of Couples After a Mastectomy or Myocardial Infarction," *Nursing Forum* 23 (1987/88): 85–91.

24. de Graaf, R., "New Treatise Concerning the Generative Organs of Women," H. B. Jocelyn and B. P. Setchell, eds., *Journal of Reproduction and Fertility*, Supplement No. 17 (1672): 103–107.

25. Gräfenberg, E., and Dickinson, R., "Conception Control by Plastic Cervix Cap," *Western Journal of Surgery, Obstetrics, and Gynecology* (1950): 337–338.

26. Kinsey Institute for Research in Sex, Gender, and Reproduction, Inc. (1998–2000), http://www.indiana.edu/-kisiss/topten.html.

27. Kreidman, E., Ph.D., *The 10-Second Kiss* (New York: Dell Publishing, 1998), 79.

28. Cole, D. A., *Seduce Me! How to Ignite Your Partner's Passion* (Universal Publishers, 2003).

Other Books from Amorata Press

The Best Sex You'll Ever Have!
Richard Emerson, $13.95
Packed with a variety of new ideas to spice up lovemaking, *The Best Sex You'll Ever Have!* illustrates risqué positions, fantasies, role playing, sex toys and erotic games.

The Little Bit Naughty Book of Sex
Dr. Jean Rogiere, $9.95
A handy pocket hardcover that is a fun, full-on guide to enjoying great sex.

Female Ejaculation: Unleash the Ultimate G-Spot Orgasm
Somraj Pokras & Jeffre Talltrees, $13.95
Opening a doorway to mind-altering sex, this how-to manual allows readers to expand their capacity for pleasure by learning to give and experience the ecstasy of female ejaculation.

The Wild Guide to Sex and Loving
Siobhan Kelly, $16.95
Packed with practical, frank and sometimes downright dirty tips on how to hone your bedroom skills, this handbook tells you everything you need to know to unlock the secrets of truly tantalizing sensual play.

To order these books call 800-377-2542 or 510-601-8301, fax 510-601-8307, e-mail ulysses@ulyssespress.com, or write to Amorata Press, P.O. Box 3440, Berkeley, CA 94703. All retail orders are shipped free of charge. California residents must include sales tax. Allow two to three weeks for delivery.

Acknowledgments

I would like to thank all the doctors, researchers, and study participants who helped me while compiling this book, with a very special thanks to Dr. Beverly Whipple for going well beyond the call of duty. Without the help of all these generous and wonderful people, this book would not exist.

About the Author

DONALD HICKS attended Southern State Community College and is the author of award-winning poetry, numerous articles, and four novels, including *The Divinity Factor* (Ozark Mountain Publishing). While writing *Unleashing Her G-Spot Orgasm*, Hicks feels blessed to have corresponded and worked with the foremost sexuality researchers of modern day.

Together with their pets, Hicks and his wife Arleta live on a rolling farm in rural Virginia, where they enjoy quiet walks, painting, gardening, and nature. He is currently working on his next novel.

To contact the author directly, e-mail him at hook books@aol.com; written correspondence can be forwarded through the publisher.